AF223796

A
WALK
ACROSS
IRELAND

Other Titles by Jonathan Wunrow & Published by *Life is Twisted Press*:

- *High Points: A Climber's Guide to Central America* (2012)
- *Adventure Inward: A Risk Taker's Book of Quotes* (2013)
- *High Points: A Climber's Guide to Central America,*
  Second Edition (2017)
- *High Points: A Climber's Guide to South America* (2018)
- *Never Stop Walking: A Wales Coast Path Adventure* (2021)
- *Paddling the Mississippi: One Story at a Time* (2022)
- *Me & Sadie, We Got Everything We Need: Stories from Paddling
  the Tennessee River* (2022)

A
WALK
ACROSS
IRELAND

JONATHAN WUNROW

Life is Twisted Press
Bloomington, IN

ISBN (Print, color edition): 978-1-7363870-8-5
ISBN (eBook): 978-1-7363870-9-2

Printed in the United States of America

Cover design by Bri Bruce Productions
Cover and Interior Photos by Jonathan Wunrow

Life is Twisted Press
801 W. 9th Street
Bloomington, Indiana 47404
Email: jonwunrow@gmail.com

A Walk Across Ireland is dedicated to my grandchildren Arlo, Rio, and Coletta who make me smile whenever I think of them. I want their Cha Cha to be an example of jumping into life, and living it to the fullest, with the hope that they will want more for themselves, and push the boundaries of what they believe they can accomplish.

That would quite literally defeat the purpose, if you stayed the same. Change is meant to be terrifying. It's meant to scare the shit out of you. No one ever grew from remaining the same. It's when that terror takes hold and you jump anyway, that's when growth occurs, that's when life rewards you.

You don't have to be an adrenaline junky to jump into life, to harness that terror. You just have to want the best for yourself. You have to respect yourself enough to want more for yourself. You have to want more than mediocre.

- Kaylee Brayne

TABLE OF CONTENTS

A
WALK
ACROSS
IRELAND

We were walking along a narrow, windy country road towards the end of our short nine-mile hike today, and it looked like rain was heading our way. So, we stopped along the side of the road, took our packs off, and fished out our raincoats.

A woman in a long winter coat came down her driveway and introduced herself. Emma asked all about our hike, and couldn't believe that we'd walked all the way from Dublin. Emma said that she and her husband had just returned home after spending the weekend in Graiguenamanagh. She described herself as a "walker"and said that someday she'd love to hike the Wicklow Way. But her husband was a farmer, and apparently not super healthy. Leslie encouraged her to find some girlfriends and do a girls' hike of the Wicklow Way.

Emma asked us about our kids and grandkids. She has four adult children. One who just returned from living in Australia for the past three years. She also has a daughter who lives in town. And her youngest is a 20-year-old boy who just got back yesterday from a trip to Spain with his buddies. And then, Emma told us about her fourth, a 28-year-old boy who died tragically last year.

Emma said, "I'm learning that you have to live your life now. It's hard to live a balanced life, but we all need to find balance in our lives, and not focus too much on work."

And then, seeming to doubt herself a little, she continued, "I think that's right, isn't it?"

Philosopher Friedrich Nietzsche, once wrote, "Enjoy Life. This is not a dress rehearsal."

Unless you believe in reincarnation, you don't get a second chance at life. You don't get a do-over. We aren't practicing in this life for the next time around. This is it. We either need to do things now, in this life, or they won't get done. And even more important to understand than the fact that this is the only life we have, is that our life . . . your life . . . my life, could end tomorrow.

Armed with the insight that, "you are only here for a short visit," as golfer Walter Hagen once noted, how are you spending your time? How are you spending your life? What are you putting off? Life is not a dress rehearsal.

In *Adventure Inward, A Risk Taker's Book of Quotes* (2014), I wrote that opportunities come to us when we open ourselves up to them, as H. Jackson Brown, Jr. said, "Opportunity dances with those on the dance floor." But you have to have the courage and determination to step onto the dance floor of life's opportunities. Do you dwell in a world of certainties and have a fear of the unknown? Are you afraid to try something new or bold, or downright outrageous? What opportunities does the dance floor hold for you?

I could write a book about the myriad excuses that we all use, at one time or another, for never doing the things we really want to do, the things we were meant to do. Too busy working. Not enough money. Too much risk. No time. Wait until the kids are out of the house. Unsupportive partner. Too old. No energy. Fear.

It took Emma a good part of her life, and the loss of her son, to get to the place where she wondered aloud to two complete strangers,whether her life had been focused too much on work, and not enough on living life now.

INTRODUCTION

My wife Leslie and I were barely finished with our 870-mile through-hike of the Wales Coast Path in 2017 when I was already dreaming about our next long-distance hike. Leslie, the more sensible of the two of us, would have nothing to do with talk of another long-distance hike after having just been away from home for two and a half months. But there is something about being on one adventure that frees my mind to dream about others.

Over the next few years, and in between through-paddling the Mississippi and Tennessee Rivers, I thought about other long-distance hikes that were in our wheelhouse—fairly easy to get to, not too strenuous, camping not a necessity, interesting people and countryside. I ended up focusing on a few: the El Camino in Spain; the North Country National Scenic Trail that transects the northern U.S. states; and the Ulster Way that travels the circumference of Northern Ireland.

In my search for our next hike, I ran across Paddy Dillon's book, *The Irish Coast to Coast Walk*, published in 1996 and now long out of print. In it, Dillon describes his hike from Dublin, heading west across Ireland for 370 miles, to Valentia Island. This route isn't the shortest way to walk across Ireland from Dublin. That would likely be Dublin straight west to Galway. But Dillon's route did string together Ireland's two most popular long-distance trails, the Wicklow Way at the beginning of his hike, and the Kerry Way at the end. And then connecting a few less-used trails across the center of the country.

Dillon's guidebook described his route as taking 21days, and averaging 17½ miles per day, for 370 total miles. His proposed hiking itinerary included three 22-mile days, and one 25-mile day. All too far for Leslie's and my 57- and 60-year-old bodies. But the idea of hiking across Ireland took root in my imagination, and I used Dillon's route as the framework to grow the plan for our own cross-Ireland hiking adventure.

The route we took ended up being 357½ miles, and took us 31 days to complete. We linked five identified trails together—Wicklow Way, South Leinster Way, East Munster Way, Blackwater Way, and Kerry Way—into one contiguous walking route from Dublin to the westernmost tip of Valentia Island. Again, this isn't the shortest way to get across Ireland, but it allowed us to do the least amount of road walking and hike what are arguably the two most scenic trails in Ireland.

Back when my son Seth and I lived on a boat in Sitka, Alaska, there was a tugboat captain named Doug, whose liveaboard was tied up a few slips further down the dock from the boat we lived on. One Saturday morning, I bought a gallon of dark purple paint that was on sale at Fleming's Paint Store with the plan to repaint the drab gray exterior of our wooden liveaboard. It wasn't until after I'd started repainting our boat purple that I realized that virtually all of the other boats in the harbor were painted either white or gray. Just as I was second guessing my frugal purchase and paint choice, Doug walked by and stopped to say good morning. I replied something like, "I'm feeling a little embarrassed about my paint choice."

Doug replied, "It doesn't matter, Jon. It's your movie."

Wise words.

Planning our hiking route across Ireland was "our movie." How much trail walking versus road walking we ended up doing, where we stayed each night, how much food and water we started out with each day, what our daily mileage would be, how far we would keep pushing despite the joint pain, bad weather, or blisters, when we would stop and enjoy the scenery and when we would keep moving . . . all were our decisions to make.

The Route

We decided to start our hike at the iconic Temple Bar Pub near the well-known Ha'Penny Bridge in Dublin, which was actually five and a half miles before the official start of the Wicklow Way in Marlay Park. We ended our hike at an old abandoned lighthouse on Bray Head at the far western tip of Valentia Island that juts out into the North Atlantic Ocean.

Our 31-day cross-Ireland hike linked together five established hiking trails. Each of the five trails we hiked have their own personality and notoriety, or lack thereof. The Wicklow Way and Kerry Way are very popular hiking trails, both because they are easily accessible from large cities and because of their incredible scenery and history. The other three trails that we hiked, to link everything together, are much less well-known and harder to find information about. We passed lots of day and weekend hikers on the Wicklow and Kerry, and virtually no one on the South Leinster, East Munster, and Blackwater trails.

Wicklow Way

The Wicklow Way is the oldest and the most scenic long-distance linear walk in Ireland. This iconic trail is 130 kilometers (81 miles) long and crosses the Wicklow Mountains from Marley Park in Dublin to Clonegal in County Carlow. The Wicklow Way is one of the most popular walks in Ireland, and is usually split into 6- or 7-day-long hiking sections. Through-hiking the Wicklow Way in a single hike is a bucket list item for lots of hikers in the U.K. and elsewhere, though we passed only a handful of Wicklow Way through-hikers during our hike. Ninety-nine percent of the hikers we passed were day-hiking one of the trail sections.

Leslie and I have decided that the new official start of the Wicklow Way should be Temple Bar Pub in Dublin rather than Marlay Park. It only seemed sensible to start a hike across Ireland at a pub.

The route is above the tree line most of the way, offering amazing views back towards Dublin and then ahead to the Wicklow Mountains. I highly recommend taking the alternate "Miner's Way" trail from Glendalough Hotel (rather than taking the official Wicklow Way route). This alternate route is about midway along the Wicklow Way, and is well worth the extra effort and slightly longer distance.

A must-read in preparation for this sections is *Walking the Wicklow Way: A Week-Long Walk from Dublin to Clonegal* (2021) by Paddy Dillon. And bring a copy with you on your hike. Dillon's hiking guidebook contains excellent maps, detailed trail descriptions, some interesting trail alternates, as well as near-the-trail lodging suggestions. Even though the Wicklow Way is well signed, having the guidebook provides interesting historic and trail information, and we did have to consult it a couple of times when we weren't sure which way to go.

We took eight days to hike what for us turned out to be 91 miles to Clonegal and the end of the Wicklow Way. Some robust through-hikers complete the trail in four or even fewer days. The extra 10 miles we walked over the official 81-mile trail included a couple of suggested trail alternates, and included having to hike off-trail to get to lodging and food.

South Leinster Way

The South Leinster Way traverses 104 kilometers (64 miles) through the heart of Ireland's farmlands, passing herds of beef cattle, dairy cows, and sheep. About half of this official trail follows narrow and relatively untraveled country roads, and the other half passes along forest tracks. The scenery is stunning in a different way than the Wicklows. Bucolic. Pastoral. Peaceful. Even though the Wicklow Way is higher, wilder, and windier, the South Leinster Way packs a lot of unexpected beauty, and is rarely traveled and even more rarely through-hiked. Despite the pasture land, there are still lots of high hills and windy open sections. I don't think we saw a single hiker during the five and a half days we were on this path.

There is no printed guidebook for the South Leinster Way. The trail officially starts in the village of Kildavin and ends in Carrick-on-Suir. A highlight of this trail is a day-long and very pleasant hike along the Barrow River.

To connect the Wicklow Way to the South Leister Way, we had to road walk from Clonegal, at the end of the Wicklow, about two and a half miles to Kildavin, where the trail sign for the start of the South Leinster Way is located. This connecting section goes up and over a few hills on a road with literally no shoulder, so watch for traffic.

What little trail information I was able to find included a couple of paragraphs that I came across when Googling the name of the trail. However, we did bring along the three 1:50,000 scale *Discovery Series* paper maps that covered the entire South Leinster Way (Sheets 68, 75, and 76). Well worth buying. The trail was generally well-marked, though some sections were overgrown and a couple of trail signs were covered up by foliage. It definitely takes some pre-planning to decide how far to hike each day on the South Leinster due to the lack of lodging options near the trail.

There is also an excellent trail map that can be found Online at https://hiiker.app/trails/ireland/county-carlow/south-leinster-way/map.

For each day's entry for the South Leinster Way, I've added a brief route description since no guidebook exists.

East Munster Way

The East Munster Way starts in the center of Carrick-on-Suir at Ormond Castle and travels 75 kilometers (45 miles) to end in Clogheen. We took four days to hike the 45 miles.

The East Munster Way is a walking route that offers lots of variety. Terrain consists mainly of forestry tracks, riverside tow paths, and quiet tarmac roads with some off-road paths that may be a little overgrown.

The trail starts in the town of Carrick-on-Suir, at the southeast extremity of County Tipperary, and follows the River Suir upstream. The Suir, held by some to be the second-longest river in Ireland, is majestic and slow moving at this point, overlooked by old castles and churches, and home to otters and herons.

At the pretty village of Kilsheelan, the route crosses into County Waterford and ascends into the foothills of the Comeragh Mountains. It soon descends again to follow the Suir into the vibrant county town of Clonmel. Leaving Clonmel, the Way crosses a western outlier of the Comeraghs to reach the northern flanks of the Knockmealdown Mountains where it meanders westward with spectacular views before descending to reach the town of Clogheen.

Once again, what little information I was able to find about this trail I got by Googling the name of the trail. We followed two

1:50,000 scale *Discovery Series* paper maps that covered the entire East Munster Way (Sheets 76 and 74). Again, well worth buying.

There is also an excellent Online map that can be found at: https://hiiker.app/trails/ireland/county-tipperary/east-munster-way.

Blackwater Way

The Blackwater Way starts in Clogheen and ends in Clonkeen. The Blackwater Way is actually a combination of two trails: Avondhu Way, 94 kilometers (57 miles) from Clogheen to Bweeng, and Duhallow Way, 67 kilometers (40 miles) that begins in Bweeng and ends in the tiny village of Clonkeen in an area referred to as "Shrone."

The Blackwater Way is a long-distance walking route in its own right that takes most hikers seven to 10 days to complete. It stretches from the borders of west County Waterford across north County Cork and into the County of Kerry. Walkers who set out along the Blackwater Way should note that accommodation options are absent over some long stretches. It may sometimes be necessary to arrange to be picked up along the route by a taxi or prearranged accommodation provider.

The Blackwater Way follows the valley of the River Blackwater. The Way is a richly varied one in terms of topography and features, and includes contouring sections along mountain flanks with great views, passing by ancient monuments such as standing stones, stone circles and cairns, and more modern monuments such as cillins (infant burial grounds) and holy wells.

Although about 28 percent of the route is on roads that carry fast traffic, the balance consists mainly of quiet tarmac roads, forestry tracks, bog roads, and moorland and field paths. Some sections can be wet and muddy in wet weather.

Since the Blackwater Way combines the older Avondhu and Duhallow Ways, hikers will encounter signs that don't always say "Blackwater."

The high point of the Blackwater Way for us was the hike through the Shrone Moore, a high, treeless and boggy area surrounded by several beautiful and barren high peaks.

Through-hikers who want to connect the Blackwater Way to the Kerry Way will need to hike about 11 and a half miles of very busy highway to get from Clonkeen to the start of the Kerry Way in Killarney.

Once again, what little trail information I was able to find about this trail, I got by Googling the name of the trail. We followed three 1:50,000 scale *Discovery Series* paper maps that covered the entire Blackwater Way (Sheets 74, 80, and 79). Again, well worth buying.

Kerry Way

The Kerry Way is Ireland's longest waymarked trail and definitely the most popular multi-day hiking trail in the Republic. Starting in the busy tourist destination of Killarney, this iconic trail loops 214 kilometers (130 miles) around the Iveragh Peninsula, and circles back to Killarney in what is a nine- to 12-day hike for most people. The Kerry Way passes through some of the most isolated and dramatic countryside in the country, following narrow country roads, forest paths, abandoned coach roads on national park land and farmland.

Cross-Ireland through-hikers will only travel the first 50 miles of the Kerry Way from Killarney to the Cahersiveen on the coast. From Cahersiveen, we hiked three miles to the Valentia Island Ferry dock, took the ferry to Knight's Town, and then hiked the final nine and a half miles of our cross-Ireland trek to Bray Head at the western tip of the island.

The four long days that it took us to hike the first 50 miles of the Kerry Way were incredibly beautiful. Even though we saw more hikers on this stretch than on any of the previous four trails, it still felt wild and remote. Virtually everyone on the Kerry Way uses a baggage transfer service. We only saw two other hikers carrying large backpacks. Because of its remote routing, the options for overnight lodging and nightly meals are pretty much pre-determined, so depending on what time of year you are hiking, you should make reservations in advance.

An essential purchase in preparing for and hiking the Kerry Way is Dónal Nolan's *The Kerry Way: A Walking Guide* (2015). This excellent guidebook offers a detailed description of the trail plus lively asides on geology, history, folklore, settlements, flora, and fauna. Above all, this guide will keep you from getting lost. The trail description is broken down into sections from the first step out of Killarney, through the high passes in the MacGillycuddy's Reeks, into the splendor of the Ring of Kerry, and back to Killarney.

Although the *Discovery Series* maps can be purchased for the Kerry Way, Nolan's guidebook has excellent maps and the trail is also very well used and well signed.

"It's Our Movie"

When we checked in at the lodge at Glenmalure, the hostess said, "Can I grab your stored bags?" I said, "No, our bags are on our backs." She seemed surprised, and said, "Well done."

Just about everyone who through-hikes the more popular Wicklow and Kerry Ways uses a baggage transfer service to move their baggage from one stop to the next each day. We did meet a small group of young, energetic hikers and passed a solo hiker on a couple of occasions on the Wicklow Way who were carrying full packs like us. But the smarter, more enjoyable and more expensive option is to hire a taxi driver or transfer service to carry the weight for you.

Of the three long-distance hikes that Leslie and I have completed in England, Wales, and now Ireland, we've yet to use a transfer service. I'm not 100 percent sure why we haven't? I've used the cost as an excuse, but to be honest I like knowing that we have everything we need on our backs . . . and it's a little more bad ass.

I have certainly made some accommodations over the years to adjust to the added physical challenges of long-distance hiking in my 50s and 60s. When I through-hiked the 2,600-mile Pacific Crest Trail in 1987, I was 25 years old. I carried an external frame pack that consistently weighed 60 to 75 pounds, depending on how many days of food we were carrying. I wore heavy leather boots with Vibram soles, and the thought of bringing hiking poles never occurred to me. I didn't have a cellphone, iPad, or charge cords because they didn't exist back them.

In contrast, our cross-Ireland hike packs were consistently around 25 to 27 pounds. Our backpacks were made of super lightweight materials with minimal internal frame staves. We both hiked in lightweight cross-trainer shoes, and carried ultra-light raincoats and down jackets that weighed six ounces each. On the Pacific Crest Trail, I carried a tent, sleeping bag, and sleeping pad that combined weighed 20 pounds. On our three long-distance hikes in the U.K. and Ireland, we ditched our tent, sleeping bag, and cooking gear for Airbnbs and hostels.

So, with age comes a bit of privilege and a lot of common sense.

Other Examples of Hiking "Our Movie"

There are lots of personal decisions to be made when planning and, hopefully, successfully completing a long-distance hike. Here are just a few for you to contemplate:

- *Bringing camping equipment, or planning the hike around indoor lodging options?* Although leaving your tent, sleeping bag and pad, stove, and cooking and eating supplies can easily drop 15 or more pounds from your load, finding an indoor place to sleep and eat at the end of a long hiking day can involve taking taxis, hitchhiking, coordinating with your host or a baggage transfer company, and/or walking quite a ways off the trail.

- *Hiking every single step of the marked trail, or doing occasional road walking and/or taking alternate routes?* There were several times, especially on the Blackwater Way, that Leslie and I decided to head off the trail and do more road walking. This was typically because there just wasn't any accessible lodging anywhere near the official route. Sometimes, the stretches of trail between lodging options or road access was 20 miles or more, which was more than we wanted to hike in a given day. For us, if we got a ride to lodging, we always made sure to get a return ride the next morning to exactly where we'd stopped walking. Our goal was to walk across Ireland from Dublin to Bray Head, and not to necessarily walk every step of the official trails that we followed.

- *Carrying electronics and power cords?* On all three of our long-distance hikes, we've chosen to carry electronics. Leslie brings her iPad, and I carry a MacBook Air laptop. We of course have our phones as well. Checking the weather, reserving lodging, staying on top of the news, and for me doing work along the way, are all things that warrant the extra weight of devices and power cords.

- *Everything else?* What types of clothing and how much? Personal hygiene items? How much food to carry? Book or no book? How much water to start the day with? Journal? How much Advil? All decisions you'll have to make either before you start hiking, or somewhere along the way. Appendix 2 provides a list of what we carried with us on this hike.

Why Go on a Long-Distance Hike?

It's the people, and the land, and the history that keeps me wanting to plan the next long-distance hike. . . . I was planning to write a bit about the people and what sets Ireland apart from other places we've traveled through. I wanted to say something about how, in many ways, Ireland is changing and evolving politically and economically, and in other ways Ireland and the Irish people have remained the same: welcoming and friendly. But I decided instead to just let you learn about these things through the pages of the book, and experience Ireland with us as we hiked along.

It's the challenge of completing something big that keeps me wanting to plan the next long-distance hike. . . . It could be ego and bragging rights that keep me motivated to go on long-distance adventures, but I want to believe that it is more about how I feel inside, in the months and years after spending weeks or months hiking or biking or paddling. Is it the desire to stand on the top of the mountain, or the sides of the mountain, that keeps me going, and the experiences along the way that make the aches and pain, and cold and rain, all worth it? One thing I do know about myself is that after standing on the summit of a big mountain, or getting to the end of a long hike, I see things differently when I get back to my normal life. I see things with "summit eyes."

It's the stories that are created that keep me wanting to plan the next long-distance hike. . . . We will all die one day. But part of me hopes that the stories I share, at least some of them, will live on.

It's the example that I want to set for my boys and my grandchildren that keeps me wanting to plan and write about the next long-distance hike or paddle or bike or climb. . . . I want to be an example of jumping into life, and living it to the fullest, with the hope that they will want more for themselves and push the boundaries of what they believe they can accomplish.

Life and death are of supreme importance.
Time passes swiftly and opportunity is lost.
Let us awaken. Do not squander your life.

- Zen Evening Chant

A WALK ACROSS IRELAND

June 16 - July 20, 2022

Ha'Penny Bridge
Dublin

Sitting at the Zanzibar Locke restaurant, waiting for the 2pm check-in time. The place is hip… modern… Leslie says, "Tribal." A cool open workspace, coffee shop, bar, and restaurant, all combined, and connected to the lobby of the Zanzibar Locke Hotel. A great spot to hang out after our long overnight flight.

Our flight arrived from Newark around 7:45am. No customs. No immigration hassles. The uniformed immigration officer asked how long we'll be in Ireland.

"Five weeks."

Her eyebrows went up.

"What are you going to be doing for five weeks?"

"We're going to hike across the country, from Dublin to Valentia Island on the southwest coast."

"Why? That doesn't sound like a vacation at all. It sounds horrible."

"We were hoping it would be fun."

"No. That's no vacation. Be safe."

Uber and Lyft are outlawed in Ireland. You can use the apps, but they just connect to a local taxi service. I actually like that. Helps keep the local taxi drivers in business.

Thomas, our taxi driver, was a fifth generation "Dub." For the entire 25-minute drive from the airport to Ha'Penny Bridge, he told us all he could about how it wasn't until the 1980s that Ireland started stepping out of the shadows and its stereotypes of being a poor and backwards country. During that time, the Irish government made public education a major focus, and gave the predominantly private Catholic education system a run for its money. The result was a generation of young people who started to lift their country up.

Thomas said that the entire country became more confident and assertive, and started asking questions, like "Why?" and "How?" and "When?" Questions that in his humble opinion, were not encouraged in the Catholic church. Thomas credited this educational revolution, combined with joining the European Union, with creating a booming economy in Ireland over the last 40 years.

Thirty-two euros for the taxi ride. I handed Thomas a 50€ note, expecting change so that I could give him a tip. He just pocketed the entire 50€ and said, "Thanks." I guess the extra was for the guided tour.

We dropped our bags at the hotel, five hours before they said we could check in, and thought about how to spend the time after having slept almost zero hours during our six-hour flight from Newark.

We got coffee in the hip cafe, and walked across the Ha'Penny walking bridge that arches over River Liffey. Thomas told us that the Vikings who came to invade Dublin in 795 AD kept on raiding and plundering, and by 840 AD there was a large Viking settlement around the area where the Zanzibar Hotel is now.

Anyway, we walked a few blocks to the Temple Bar Pub where we'll officially start our hike tomorrow. (It wasn't until later in the day that I found out why the seemingly redundant words "bar" and "pub" are both in the same name). And then we walked along the south side of the Liffey River for a mile or so towards the port and the sea. And then back up the north side of the river. It was nice to just be out walking and absorbing this more modern part of Dublin.

After months of planning, it seems weird that we'll start our cross-Ireland hike tomorrow morning!

We met a super red-faced Dub during our walk along the Liffey who, over the course of 10 minutes, convinced us that he's an anti-immigrant, probably racist Donald Trump lover who dreams about the old days when only Irish people lived in Ireland. He said that most of the places you go to visit in Ireland don't have Irish people anymore. He also complained about the fact that some Ukrainians have arrived in Dublin to flee the Russian attack on Ukraine that is now in its 110th day.

The very red-faced gentleman literally said, "Why don't they just go to the other side of their own country to get away from the war? Why do they have to come to my country?"

Anyway, this guy turned us on to the information that Northern Ireland just elected a Sinn Féin leader. Sinn Féin is the party that has been linked to the paramilitary Irish Republican Army that has been trying to get Northern Ireland out of the grip of the United Kingdom for centuries. It is the first time in 700 years (according to this guy) that Northern Ireland will not be ruled by a backer of the United Kingdom.

Sinn Féin's main platform is supporting a united Ireland, the unification of Northern Ireland with the Republic of Ireland. I just Googled the topic, and this Sinn Féin victory, is "the first time an Irish Nationalist Party has had the majority since Northern Ireland was founded as a Protestant State in 1921."

So, I'm planning to watch the news over the next few weeks. This red-faced, anti-immigrant Dub seemed to support a unified Ireland. As I'd guess most people in the Republic of Ireland do. I'll find out.

We checked into our room at 2:30pm, spread our shit all over the place, showered, and were napping before 3pm. We decided that a two-hour nap would be our limit.

Walking back over the Ha'Penny Bridge and the River Liffey, we planned to grab a beer at the iconic Temple Bar Pub. I had been wondering why a place that served alcohol was called both a "bar" and a "pub?" It seemed a little redundant. But the "bar" of Temple Bar refers to the location of this pub, in an area known as Temple Bar. This river shoreline area was built up (creating a sand/land "bar") to create a place for gardens of the rich folks who lived in the area, including the Temple family. So, the iconic pub, owned incidentally by U2 band members Bono and The Edge, is known as the pub in the neighborhood of Temple Bar, or the Temple Bar Pub.

There you have it!

Anyway, when we got there, it was absolutely jam packed with people, and we were hungry and ready for our first pint of Guinness, so we took a few photos and wandered on to busy Dame Street a few blocks away. It was the end of a Thursday workday, so there were lots of people stopping off for a beer. We settled on Bo-Bo's

Burgers. The Guinness was smoother and creamier than I remembered. I told the lady behind the bar that a Guinness in Dublin tastes way better than an Guinness in the U.S.

Leslie and I both wanted seafood for dinner since we'll start walking away from the sea tomorrow. We stumbled upon Quays, a restaurant that didn't look like much from the street, but once we walked up the stairs to this second floor restaurant we realized that it was packed. By the time we left, there were at least 50 people lined up to get in. Fresh mussels, amazing fish chowder, and grilled salmon! All really, really good.

Leslie is already in bed, and I'm on my way. We have probably slept a total of four hours in the past 36. Great day in Dublin. It's hard to believe that we just arrived this morning.

Tomorrow we throw on our packs and hike!

Hiking Day #1
Temple Bar Pub to Pine Forest Art Center - 12.5 Miles

"Stop along the way and get a fucking shrink."

Definitely the quote of the day. This was from our taxi driver, Robbie, who picked us up at the end of our first day of hiking. He was taking us to the seaside village of Bray, where our hotel is tonight, since there was no lodging near where we ended up.

Robbie had just finished making several very supportive comments like, "You had a bang-on hike today," and "You should feel proud of yourselves for such a great first day." He was asking where we planned to hike to tomorrow, and then the next day. I couldn't quite remember the names of the places, but Robbie helped fill in the blanks since he's lived nearby in Enniskerry his entire life, and spent much of it "tramping through the hills with his mates."

I ended up telling Robbie that we planned to hike all the way to the west coast of Ireland.

"To where then?"

"To Valentia Island, right to the tip."

"All the way? Make sure you stop along the way to get a fucking shrink."

Robbie continued, "You'll be able to tell your friends back in American that you walked across an entire country."

Robbie said that a lot of Irish speak fluent Gaelic. Including himself. "It doesn't do any good in Europe, knowing Gaelic, but it gives me pride in being Irish. I'm glad I know how to speak it."

During our ride I mentioned to Robbie that we'd also hiked the entire coast of Wales.

"I hate Wales," he shot back.

"You hate Wales?"

"Aye. I can't understand them when they talk. Not a word."

That was funny, since we were having a hell of a time understanding Robbie.

Robbie told us that we needed to walk down to the seashore and have dinner at the Harbour Bar. He said we absolutely had to go. So, we did. It's a great old bar near the waterfront in Bray. Lots of outside picnic tables. The food comes out in a small cardboard box. The entire menu consisted of just battered and fried fresh fish and chips, and a fish burger. And they both came with a mountain of thick chips.

I'd promised myself no alcohol tonight, or I'd be sound asleep by 7pm. But I ended up getting a pint of Guinness that went down especially well. Leslie got a glass of white wine. This particular Guinness almost had a blackberry flavor to it. No carbonation, as usual, but it tasted sweet and berry-like. Very different than any Guinness I've ever had, including yesterday.

I just Googled, "Does Guinness taste different in Irish pubs?" and found out that the Guinness served in Ireland is actually "scientifically proven to taste better than elsewhere." It's not only the ambiance of drinking it in Ireland, but the fact that it is fresher, and that pubs in Ireland know how to properly store and, more importantly, pour a pint of Guinness. What I read did not account for the berry flavor that I could have sworn I tasted.

Okay. Hiking. We actually did complete the first day of our hike across Ireland today.

Twelve and a half miles. Not bad. But our legs are achy and tired tonight. Especially after we walked the 15 minutes uphill back to the Firefly Hotel, with our bellies full of Harbour Bar fish, chips, and beer.

We decided that the unofficial start of the Wicklow Way, the first trail we'd be following out of Dublin, should be the Temple Bar Pub instead of the trail's official start at Marlay Park. So, after packing up this morning, and grabbing breakfast and coffee, we put on our packs and walked back over the Ha'Penny Bridge and River Liffey one final time and straight to Temple Bar Pub. We asked an employee if he'd take our picture out front of the bright red bar to mark the official start of our adventure.

It was five and a half miles through the streets of Dublin to Marlay

Park. It was fun to walk through the morning hustle and bustle of the big city, with double decker buses passing us, and people heading off to work. At one point we passed a school yard and about 50 middle school kids were lined up, each standing in a gunny sack in a long, straight line waiting for the starting bell. And then we stood and watched most of them fall over, one-by-one, before they reached the race's halfway point. Year-end field day.

We had a little lunch at a café in Marlay Park. There was some kind of construction and setting up of bleachers and a stage, that I found out later was for the "Hella-Mega Tour," a huge outdoor concert featuring Weezer and Green Day. Big names.

There were barricades set up all over, directing foot traffic around the massive concert area, so we never actually found the official start of the Wicklow Way. We just started walking down an asphalt path that we were sure was the right way, and that turned out to not be the start of the trail.

Funny.

We got lost right out of the gate. I had to eventually use the map on my phone to figure out where we'd gone wrong and how to get to the actual trail.

At the opposite end of the park, we met an older guy, a walker, who said he'd hiked several sections of the Wicklow Way over the years, and was excited to hear about our hike. Its' nice to not be in a hurry, with time to stop and talk for five minutes.

The guy pointed out which way we needed to go to follow the trail out of the park, and explained the right and left turns we'd be negotiating up ahead.

After thanking him for his kindness, we headed off and immediately took a wrong turn. I heard this car honking behind us, and turned around to see this same guy driving towards us and pointing us in the right direction.

Lost twice in the first mile of the official trail.

About a mile out of the park, the Wicklow Way heads up a steep hill on a very narrow road, and then turns left into Kilmashogue Forest, and then onto a dirt path at about mile seven for the day. And then up, up, up. Three miles straight up. This was miles eight through 10, so our legs were getting pretty wobbly and tired.

We were treated to great views looking back at Dublin and the ocean behind us, with plenty of heather and gorse and bilberry along the trail above the tree line. We were finally back up in the hills. It was a warm day for June in Ireland, maybe 70 degrees, but clouds and a constant breeze made for perfect hiking weather.

We passed around a dozen hikers coming towards us, down the hill, including two with big backpacks. And as we rested at one point, a solo hiker with a big pack passed us from behind, saying he just "threw a few things in his bag, and decided to head to Clonegal" (the end of the Wicklow Way).

Then downhill two miles on throbbing knees and hips, to a narrow road (R116) and Pine Forest Art Center. I didn't have any cell service at the spot we'd planned to stop for the day, so I walked to a house down the driveway of the art center, to ask if they could call a taxi for us.

A very apprehensive woman eventually answered the door, and while never taking the chain lock off the door, agreed to call a taxi, as we talked through the three-inch opening. She warily said she'd never called a taxi from her house before. Next time I'll bring Leslie with me when I knock on a stranger's door in the middle of nowhere.

Day one is in the books!! Leslie just said, "It sort of feels like we never stopped hiking from our Wales trip, and this is just the next section."

Day #2
Pine Forest Art Center to Crone House Car Park – 10.2 Miles
Total – 22.7 Miles

We lost the trail two more times today. We're a little out of practice, I guess? Definitely not giving the impression that we are seasoned long-distance hikers. Yesterday, both wrong turns happened in the first mile of the trail. Today, we missed a trail turn-off two more times. First, coming down from Prince William's Seat, a high point that we didn't take the extra time to hike a side trail to the top of. Coming down off the other side, we were on a bit of a gravel "road" and missed the trail cutting off to the left, and just kept on the gravel road for a good mile. We ended up coming out at the right spot, a car park at Curtlestown Wood.

At the parking area, there were two day-hikers ready to hike up to Prince William's Seat. They asked us if the trail they were starting on was the right one, since they saw us with backpacks coming in from a different (wrong) direction. We definitely weren't the right people to ask.

Leslie and I both agreed that we need to pay better attention both to the guidebook, *Walking the Wicklow Way,* that I'm carrying and rarely referring to, and to the small trail signs that are sometimes hidden amidst tall ferns.

And then it wasn't more than an hour after we'd decided to pay better attention that we stopped to sit on a pile of logs to eat some lunch. When we got up to head out again, we continued following a wide gravel back road, and walked right past our trail turn, and just kept on the gravel path all the way downhill to a river, where the gravel road ended. We scouted all over for a trail along the river, but couldn't find anything. Twice in one hour.

Rather than hike back up the hill to retrace our steps, we took an overgrown path along the creek and through the forest, figuring we'd meet up with the trail eventually. Which we did, about a quarter mile upriver.

So . . . we REALLY need to pay better attention as we're walking and then remember what I read in the trail description. Knowing that the Wicklow Way is one of the most popular hiking trails in Ireland has me lulled into not paying close attention.

It's a Saturday, and there were lots of people on the trail today. We saw three or four folks with bigger packs on, and a couple with rolled up sleeping pads. We also passed a group of Boy Scouts on a day hike, and a group of teenagers coming out of the woods looking like they'd spent the night.

Around mile two this morning on the way up to Prince William's Seat, which again we never really saw, we passed the finish line for a trail race. There were tents and cars and flags. And an official electronic finish line timer, with a guy sitting in a little booth with a laptop. It was around 11am, and the organizers said the race was almost done.

Later in the day, we saw two older women and a really, really old guy on a day hike. The guy could easily have been 100 years old. He reminded me of my dad in his later years, all hunched over with a cane in one hand and a hiking pole in the other. Good for them, being out here hiking on a Saturday.

The trail was all ups and downs today. Just a little flat section as it ran along the river for half a mile or so. And the trail took on several different personalities. Gravel road, paved road, dirt path, grassy meadow, rocky trail, and one section of steep downhill made of huge rock steps.

The weather was cooler today. And overcast. Highs were only around 58 degrees, so with a breeze it was chilly when we stopped for a break and our sweat started to cool. We're into the Wicklow Mountains now. Worn down ridges and peaks with names like Great Sugar Loaf, Knockree, Tibradden Mountain, and Hill of Howth.

Six and a half miles from our start at Pine Forest Art School was the massive Knockree Hostel, just a few hundred yards off the trail. This huge hostel is the most common stopping point on day one of the Wicklow Way, but has been closed for three years due to the pandemic. And closed for all of this year (2022) as well.

We started our day today by walking to Starbucks in Bray, and then to the SuperValu grocery store to buy food for lunch. My legs felt stiff and sore from our first day out yesterday. Leslie says that her feet are sore. Frank picked us up in his taxi to take us back to the spot we stopped yesterday. He was super funny. He said that our driver from yesterday afternoon, Robbie, "hates everything" when I mentioned that he didn't like Wales.

We talked with Frank about Northern Ireland politics as we headed from the coast, back into the hills. And about Sinn Féin winning the most seats in the Assembly. Frank said he thinks that 85 percent of the people in the Republic favor a unified Ireland. Apparently Sinn Féin is a popular political party here in the Republic of Ireland as well.

Beautiful hiking day.

Part of the trail was along a river. We also had some great hilltop views out to the ocean. And lots of walking in the forest. Our hike ended at the Crone House Car Park. Still 1.8 miles from the

Coolakay B&B, where I'd made a reservation for the night. We assumed we'd have to walk that additional distance, so we already had it in our heads that it'd be a 10.2-mile day.

There was a sign in the parking lot to call Coolakay for a pick up, but Leslie insisted that we walk the extra 1.8 miles since it was already part of the plan this morning. She's bad ass when it comes to completing what she's set out to do.

It was one mile downhill and then half a mile up a very steep road, and then were there. I took lots of pictures of horses, cows, sheep, and tractors along the way to send to our two-year-old grandson, Arlo.

After a shower and a nap, we caught a taxi ride with John into the cute little village of Enniskerry. I wanted to go to a little Italian restaurant called Emelia's. It was booked, so we went next door to the Enniskerry Inn, which was also a nice place, and also booked. But they squeezed us in. I think Enniskerry must be a popular spot for people from Dublin to come to on the weekends.

Good food. Good beer. I had a hard time standing up after dinner. My right hip is sore, and my legs were really tired. Leslie said my eyes looked exceptionally tired, too.

No place to get ice cream in Enniskerry, so we called John and got a ride back to the Coolakay.

Great day. Tomorrow we start by going three miles straight uphill!

Day #3
Crone House Car Park to Wicklow Way Lodge B&B – 11.5 Miles
Total – 34.2 Miles

Today was full of variety. Various types of trail. Various types of weather. Various types of scenery. Varied winds. A lot packed into a single day. And it was our hardest hiking day of our first three days. It started with about five miles of consistent uphill from the Crone House Car Park to just below the top of Djouce Peak.

I didn't sleep very well last night. My muscles were achy, and I had a dry sore throat. And even a bit of a stomachache. "Suffering from continuous dull pain" is how the dictionary describes "achy." I totally thought I might be coming down with COVID. I should've taken a few Advil to help me sleep.

Breakfast at Coolakay B&B was great. Options included a full Irish breakfast, or made-to-order eggs, bacon, or whatever we wanted. Plus, an array of fruit, yogurt, and cereal. It was good, but reminded us of every breakfast we had on our 73-day hike around the coast of Wales a couple of years ago.

Yvonne, the owner, took our orders and then bustled around. She and her husband, who are also sheep farmers and maintain a museum of old farm machinery including more than 60 tractors, have been running Coolakay for the past 21 years.

A taxi picked us up at 9am to bring us back to the car park where we left off yesterday, and we were hiking by 9:30am. Today, I took extra special care to keep a better eye on the trail guide descriptions, the map, and the trail signs. (And I'm pleased to announce that we did NOT take a single wrong turn today!)

The trail passed through pine and poplar forests, while climbing continuously for five miles. It was exhausting with our 30-plus-pound packs. Which doesn't sound like much weight, until you remember that you are 60 years old, and are heading uphill for a few hours straight on sore legs.

There were lots of day hikers out today. Sunday. Father's Day in Ireland and in the U.S. But we didn't see anyone carrying more than daypacks today. Walkers from both directions hike this section of the Wicklow Way to get to the top of Djouce Peak, the highest point on this multi-day trail.

Right as the trail climbed out of the trees and above the tree line, we passed Powerscourt Waterfall cascading down below us to the left. At 400 feet high, Powerscourt is the second highest waterfall in Ireland. Above the tree line where we were hiking, the wind starting picking up, and it was windy and chilly for the next few hours. We were both tired, and wanted to take a break and eat the lunches that Yvonne had packed, but it was too cold and windy, so we trudged on . . . and on . . . and on.

We rounded Djouce Peak and then up and over the other side of White Hill, and then dropped down into a forested area where we crawled on our hands and knees into a densely packed grove of trees to get out of the wind. It wasn't until we'd taken off our packs, that we realized we weren't the first hikers to head off the trail and take cover at this spot. There was used toilet paper everywhere, and lots of evidence of toilet breaks from the last few years.

My back was soaked with sweat, along with the windbreaker I was wearing. We both dug out warmer jackets from our packs so that we didn't freeze while we ate our ham and cheese sandwiches with crisps and an apple.

It was really beautiful up high on the trail today. A few grazing sheep dotting the hillsides. Other than the cold wind, it was a perfect hiking day. On the way down the other side, we stopped for a photo at a large boulder with "J. B. Malone" carved into it. Apparently, J. B. was responsible for establishing the Wicklow Way, having first proposed the idea in 1966.

Heading down, and then down some more, we saw Lough Tay, a lake nestled beneath a mountain ridge that had several wooden A-frame structures and two long docks at one end. I thought it looked like a small resort with cabins, but we found out later that this was one of the filming sites for the mini-series *Vikings*, which we loved and was mostly filmed in this part of Ireland.

Through the afternoon, it got warmer as we dropped out of the mountains and the sun came out. Low 60s and sunny is plenty hot for me. The trail followed a road past some large stone gates and a car park, and above another road that led down to a huge mansion, owned by the Guinness family.

We ended up hiking through forests and fields, above the village of Roundwood, and on to Wicklow Way Lodge, located literally right along the official hiking route. Very convenient.

The owners of Wicklow Way Lodge are Marilyn and her husband Seamus. And, lordy, Marilyn was a talker. We stood and visited with her for quite a while, more than ready to be off our aching feet and legs. Both of us were sweaty and stinky, and dying for a shower and to just sit down.

Marilyn told us that Matthew McConaughey had stayed here twenty years ago. And she told us all about the filming of *Vikings*, and how the actor who played Ragnar would hang out in the pubs in nearby Roundwood.

We got a taxi into Roundwood and had dinner at the Coach House. After dinner we bought cookies and milk at a little local market and sat at a picnic table devouring our dessert.

Leslie realized when we were unpacking our bags this afternoon that she'd left her iPad at Coolakay B&B. So, Marilyn contacted

Yvonne to arrange for a taxi driver to drive it over to us for the small fee of 40 euros.

Its 8:35pm. Time for bed. We both rinsed our socks, undies, and T-shirts, and hung them outside to hopefully dry overnight. Tomorrow is a short mileage day, and we are both looking forward to it. We're thinking of it as a day off, even though we'll still be hiking seven and a half miles or so. Today was only day three, and our aching bodies aren't used to hiking in the hills with backpacks . . . yet.

Day #4
Wicklow Way Lodge B&B to Glendolough Lodge – 8 Miles
Total – 42.2 Miles

We're sitting outside by a creek next to The Barn at the Glendolough Hotel. It's a café/bistro kind of place, attached to the historic hotel. A beautiful park setting next to the Monastic City, a popular tourist attraction in the Wicklow Mountains complete with tour buses and large groups of people speaking languages like Italian and German.

It's a little after 4pm and we've already had a shower and nap! We grabbed deli sandwiches, Pringles, and apples at a little food market in nearby Laragh. So, along with my Smithwick Red Ale and Leslie's St. Kevin's Red, we're having ourselves a proper afternoon picnic!

The sky has been cloudless all day!

Cloudless in Ireland!

And the high was around 70 degrees. An absolutely beautiful day for hiking and for picnicking.

We had a very short hiking day today. The next stopping spot is in Drumgoff, 10 miles away. In planning out the first few days of this hike, months ago, Day 4 was always going to be a short one. We'll make up for it over the next few days.

We had a great breakfast this morning and then packed and walked out the front door of the Wicklow Way Lodge by 9am and onto the "trail," which at this point is a narrow tarmac country lane. I had my first "Full Irish" breakfast of the trip: one fried egg, two finely ground sausages, two slices of fried red pudding (blood sausage), and two pieces of ham with lots of sautéed mushrooms and two small sautéed tomatoes. I have a hard time getting over the thought of red pudding consisting of ground up pork mixed with blood, and then stuffed in sausage casings and pan-fried. But it didn't taste too bad, actually.

We started our breakfast with Marilyn's "famous" porridge, which was pretty damn good. It consisted of cooked oats with lots of brown sugar and heavy cream. Orange juice. Coffee. Definitely a proper breakfast.

Our short hike today started by climbing a steep country lane up and over several step stiles (wooden steps that go up one side and down the other side of a stone wall or fence) that are usually built to get around locked farmer's gates. We hiked around some farmer's fields, up over Paddock Hill, and then down the other side.

Leslie tried to shoot a short video of me trying to sneak up on some sheep to send to our grandson Arlo, but they ran away and the video was a bust. I settled for one photo of sheep and a second photo of sheep poop to send to our Arlo, who is obsessed with farm animals and tractors.

A cloudless sky all day today. At one point, I said, "This has to be the best day in the history of Ireland!"

We walked into the little village of Laragh before noon, and stopped to buy some groceries for dinner tonight and lunch tomorrow. We were definitely in no rush today, so we sat outside the store and ate a pint of fresh local strawberries and a Diet 7UP while we tried to find room in our completely stuffed backpacks for the food we'd just purchased.

When we got to Glendalough Hotel, we were too early to check in, so we dropped off our packs and went for a short walk to check out the nearby Monastic City. I don't quite get the "city" part, but there was a big stone church that was built sometime between 900 and 1200 AD, a 100-foot-tall stone bell tower that was also over 1,000 years old, and a cemetery full of gravestones that were so weathered that we couldn't read many of the dates. We did see some that in the mid-1700s.

Leslie is always intrigued by old cemeteries. She likes to see how old people were when they died, and feels especially sad when she sees the graves of small children, even if they died 250 years ago. It brought back memories of walking through similar cemeteries during our long-distance hikes in Wales and England.

I wanted to walk a ways further to check out our route for tomorrow. The signage seemed confusing, heading away from the hotel. We're going to take an "alternate route" for the first five miles tomorrow morning, and I wanted to make sure I knew where the turnoff is. It's supposed to rain tomorrow, so I'd rather get lost finding the route today than tomorrow morning.

It was a beautiful walk around a small lake and then up to a second lake that we'll walk around tomorrow.

The days are long in Ireland in mid-June. It seems like it's light until 10:30pm, and daylight again at 4am. We really haven't seen night time in Ireland yet.

A spectacular day! Nice to have a shorter hiking day to give our leg muscles and knees and calves a bit of a rest.

Day #5
Glendolough Lodge to Glenmalure Lodge in Drumgoft
10 Hard Miles; Total – 52.2 Miles

Today we started the day by hiking an identified Wicklow Way alternate route on "Miner's Way" and through Van Diemen's Land. Definitely a good decision.

It is very unusual for us to walk even a few steps farther than we have to on a long-distance hike. Usually we get our walking done for the day, and then lay in our beds until the next day. There were 100 sites that we never saw that were only a quarter or half a mile off the Wales Coast Path or South West Coast Path, points of interest that we never hiked to because of the extra distance it added to our already long hiking days. So the fact that we hiked an extra two and a half miles yesterday to check out the area around Glendolough Lodge and took a longer alternate route today that added a mile and a quarter and some additional uphill hiking is pretty unprecedented for us.

The alternate route, Miner's Way, was well worth the extra mileage. The scenery, especially as we climbed above the Glendolough Upper Lake, was absolutely stunning! And the predicted rain never came.

As we hiked up above Upper Lake, we saw lots of red deer, sheep, and even some goats along the boulder-strewn sides of the valley as the trail climbed, and climbed, and climbed.

Today was one of those days when I said out loud, "You don't get to see this amazing scenery unless you're willing to put in the work to get there."

Our first three miles were flat as we walked around the Lower and Upper Lakes. Then the trail climbed for a good two miles up a fairly steep and rocky trail. Every few minutes we stopped and turned around to take in the views (and to catch our breath).

At the end of Upper Lake, and where the steeper uphill section started, were the remains of several mines and collapsed stone buildings from the mid-1800s. I read that about 60 men, women, and children lived up here at the mine year round. They mined primarily for lead, but also for silver and zinc.

No one was on the trail this morning. We had our hotel buffet breakfast at 8:15am, and were hiking just after 9am. It was nice to have the trail to ourselves.

At the top of the first of two long climbs, we took off our packs and laid in the grass as sheep and deer watched us rest.

Since first reading about this alternate route on the Wicklow Way a few days ago, I'd been looking forward to getting to this spot: Van Diemen's Land. My favorite band, U2, has a song by the same name on the *Rattle and Hum* album. U2 guitarist, The Edge, wrote the lyrics and sings the song on the album.

Because of the U2 connection, knowing that we'd be hiking to Van Diemen's Land was exciting for me. We got up there and I took several photos of the barren and desolate area where an old mine was located. I was planning to send the photos to my son Seth, since we've gone to a couple of U2 concerts together . . . "Dad is at the famous Van Diemen's Land of U2 fame."

Then . . . I read the lone interpretive sign, posted by some building ruins near where we'd stopped for a break. I learned that the real Van Diemen's Land is actually the name that was given to what is now known as Tasmania. And this mining area in Ireland was named Van Diemen's Land Mine because it was so remote and desolate, like the real island south of Australia.

So . . . U2 did not write a song about this place after all. The Edge wrote it about John Boyle O'Reilly, the leader of an 1864 Irish uprising against England after the great famine. He was arrested and banished to the Australian state of Tasmania.

I never did send that email to Seth.

There was a small river with several waterfalls coming down alongside the trail as we climbed this morning. At one particularly waterfally spot, I refilled my water bottle. We were quickly drinking what we had, and were not even half way done with our day's hike. I knew that there were sheep and deer in the area, and there was a chance that the water had Giardia, so I collected it where it was really moving fast, and not sitting stagnant. I was worried about hiking with no water for the rest of the day, and decided to risk it.

Fingers crossed that we both don't end up with projectile diarrhea!

We stopped for lunch on the trail just as it started heading downhill. We made sandwiches from the meat, cheese, and bread we bought yesterday in Laragh. A beautiful spot for a lunch break.

And then it was down, down, down. First on a trail, and then on old logging roads. My legs were really starting to ache those last few miles. At one point, I convinced myself that we'd missed a turnoff and had gone too far on the logging road. So, we both backtracked several hundred yards until we found a trail marker that assured us we were okay. After losing the trail a few times in our first two days, I wasn't in the mood to miss another turnoff.

We made it to Glenmalure Lodge around 2:45pm. There were several picnic tables outside and people drinking their pints of Guinness. We took our packs off and went into the old traditional Irish pub to order a couple of different kinds of very refreshing ciders. So good after a day of backpacking.

Neither of us wanted to move from the picnic table. We just enjoyed being off our feet and being done for the day. Leslie says it's her favorite time of the day—the moment when we are done hiking and know our work is done for the day. And we feel proud of ourselves and our accomplishment. No thought about tomorrow.

It was an exceptionally hard 10 miles today. We didn't see many other hikers, and the few we saw were all carrying day packs.

When we checked in at the Glenmalure, the hostess said, "Can I grab your stored bags from our store room?" I said, "No, our bags are on our backs." She seemed surprised, and said, "Well done." More confirmation that most people who hike the Wicklow Way use a transfer service to get their luggage from one spot to another.

Not us!!

Day #6
Glenmalure Lodge to Kyle's Farmhouse B&B - 15 Miles
Total – 67.2 Miles

What sticks out the most in my mind about today's 15-mile hike is . . . we hiked 15 miles up two big hills and one smaller one, and the fucking flies! We were followed by a hoard of obnoxious flies the entire day! There were a few moments when we were up high on a barren mountainside, and there was enough of a breeze to keep the flies away. But the other 97 percent of the time dozens of flies were constantly buzzing around my head, into my ears, in my eyes. Super annoying, and bad enough to get me to think evil thoughts. There were times I could make one swat with my right hand and kill four or five flies all at once.

The flies made stopping for breaks pretty miserable, too. Short breaks, and a short lunch stop.

But we cranked out 15 miles through the Wicklow Mountains. We knew in advance that it would be a long, hard day. And it was. We left the Glenmalure Lodge just before 9am and got to Kyle's Farmhouse B&B around 3:45pm totally pooped but very happy.

We actually hiked a little bit off and on with four youngsters, younger than our kids (maybe mid to late 20s?). They started this morning in Glendolough at 5:30am! And were to Glenmalore by 8:30am, which is where we started this morning. They already had about eight and a half miles in before we even started.

Pretty hard core.

We passed each other back and forth through the day, and shared a lunch stop together. Lee, Li, Daniel, and his younger sister Niamh. Niamh was the trip planner and organizer. They are hiking the Wicklow Way in five days. We are taking eight days. They are moving right along and hiking lots more miles every day than we are. And they're carrying tents, sleeping bags, and cooking gear.

Youth.

At one point today, Daniel said of Niamh, "She's like the French Foreign Legion," because she just goes and goes. It was Niamh's idea for them to hike 23-plus miles today. And they got it done by 4pm! All four are staying at the same place we are tonight, at Kyle's Farmhouse B&B, but they camped the last two nights.

By the way, Niamh is pronounced "Neeve."

Today's hike was mostly through forests, but we did get some great views along the way, both of the Wicklows and looking west into the interior "plains" of Ireland.

We had Glenmalure pack us a lunch for today. A pretty tasty ham, cheese, and "salad" sandwich with a candy bar and bottle of water. Margaret, the Farmhouse B&B owner, gave us a ride into Tinahely this evening so we could get dinner. We're eating at Pub-O'Conner's. I had a pepperoni pizza and a side of broccoli, and Leslie had a Cajun chicken burger with chips. A Guinness for me and a Pinot Grigio for Leslie.

When we first showed up at the B&B, Margaret offered us each an ice-cold 16-ounce Southwick Lager. We set our packs down, before even going inside, and sat at her patio chairs and table and enjoyed the fact that we accomplished what we'd set out to do today.

Sometimes that's good enough. Just to accomplish what you set out to do.

I walked with Daniel for about 45 minutes today. And he asked me why I do things like long-distance hiking, biking, canoing, and mountain climbing.

I said that I almost never do two- to three-day trips, or weekend trips. Like never. I want to do something at least long enough so that when I throw my pack on my back, it feels like it belongs there. That I've been paddling long enough that it feels like the paddle belongs in my hands, and that paddling is the most normal motion that I could do.

Daniel asked, "How long does that take? How long to get to that point?"

"Two weeks? Ten to 14 days?" It takes that long for my mind and my body to find that groove where what I'm doing feels like breathing. Natural. Normal.

Today was Day 6. I'm not in the groove yet.

Day #7
Kyle's Farmhouse B&B to Boley Bridge and Central House B&B –
14 Miles
Total – 81.2 Miles

Sean says his "B&B" stands for "Bed and Beer."

Last night we told Margaret that we were planning to walk across Ireland. She said that she meets one or two people a year that are planning to hike across the country. So, they're out there. But we won't likely meet any of them.

As a matter of fact, during our 14-mile hike today from Kyle's B&B to the little village of Shellalagh, we didn't see any other hikers other than the youngsters.

We're sitting outside at a picnic table at Parkview House with two pints of ice-cold Bulmer's Irish cider. It has an orange tint to it. So nice to be done with our hiking today.

It was our longest hiking day yet. We left Kyle Farmhouse around 9:15am and got to Boley Bridge, our stopping point, at around 4:15pm. Twelve miles, 14 miles, 15 miles . . . they are all long days when hiking through the mountains. And with a 30-plus pound pack and non-stop ups and downs, we're usually pretty exhausted two-thirds of the way through the day, no matter how far we're hiking. The final few miles are always hard.

We're at a point in this hike (similar to past hikes), on hiking Day 7, when our feet are starting to show signs of wear. We're both developing small blisters on our toes, and the bottom of Leslie's feet have really started to ache. Just a throbbing ache that Advil doesn't seem to have an impact on.

We started our day with a smashing breakfast, made to order by Margaret. Our four new hiking friends (we've started calling them "the kids") were already downstairs having breakfast when we came down. We started hiking before they headed out this morning, and they caught up to us around mile eight.

Leslie and I decided to take the "Kyle Loop" option to start the day. It takes off straight uphill from the farmhouse, rather than heading a half-mile back down the hill to the trail junction at Sandyford Bridge.

The Kyle Loop option heads uphill for the first mile. My legs hadn't fully recovered from yesterday's 15 miles, so as Leslie bolted ahead, I just plodded along, dropping further and further behind.

There was a big wind farm with several giant power generating windmills at the top of Ballycumber Hill. The flies were atrocious again today. Just clouds of them hovering around our faces and ears. They definitely like my sweat more than Leslie's.

The first half of the hike today was on nice, narrow grassy paths. We didn't see any other hikers other than the kids all day. The further from Dublin we go, the fewer people we see on the trail.

We saw lots of horses, and cows, and tractors today. I shot several videos of tractors driving on roads and fields, and emailed them to my grandson Arlo. I also shot videos of Leslie feeding two horses and of a couple of donkeys that came up pretty close to us.

Seeing all the farm animals helped break up the hiking. I think that's the reason it took us over seven hours to hike 14 miles. Lots of stops to talk with and photograph horses and donkeys.

All day long we'd been looking forward to walking past Tallon's

Pub, also known as The Dying Cow, a very small pub literally in the middle of nowhere. But it's mentioned in our Wicklow Way guidebook, and John the lorry driver told us yesterday that we had to stop into The Dying Cow.

Drinking alcohol and then hiking is never a great idea, but we figured with only hour and a half miles to go for the day, we could handle it.

About a mile before we got to The Dying Cow, the kids hiked up behind us, so all six of us walked together the last 30 minutes to the pub.

The pub itself is tiny on the inside, but had lots of picnic tables outside. I'd already heard the story two or three times of how the pub's name came to be. But I couldn't resist asking the very, very old and very nice lady behind the bar to tell the story, which basically goes like this . . .

> *Over a hundred years ago, it was illegal to sell alcohol on Sundays. But one particular Sunday, there were about a dozen local guys at Tallon's having a drink. The local police caught wind of this, and came in and arrested the lady owner. She explained to the police that she wasn't selling any alcohol at all. But, rather, she had a very sick cow who was dying, and these nice neighbors had come over to help her with her dying cow. And the only way she could repay their kindness, was with beer. Well, apparently they arrested her anyway, and all twelve of the neighbors went down to testify that what she'd said about the cow was true, so the police let her go. And as the story goes, the lady didn't even own a cow.*

After the story, we sat outside with the kids and I bought a round of beer for everyone. We talked a bit about where we were all from and what was going on in our lives. It was fun to get to know them all a little bit better.

We hiked on to Boley Bridge, a few miles outside of Shillellagh, and called Phil, the owner of Central House, for a ride to his B&B. He'd inherited this few-hundred-year-old building in the center of town, and was devoting himself to renovating the bedrooms. It was a great place to spend the night, and close to the post office and local food market.

The satisfaction of being done for the day is hard to describe. But on long-distance hiking days like today, when the highs aren't terribly high and the lows aren't very low, taking off your backpack and smelly shoes, taking a shower, resting, eating, reading, and journaling, are all things that bring joy.

We've been sitting in bed for the last hour or so, planning out our next few days after we finish the Wicklow Way and start the South Leinster Way. We don't have a guidebook for this next trail, because there isn't one. But I have two different sets of maps that I downloaded from the Internet. So, we're sitting here with me on my laptop, and Leslie on her iPad, and paper maps spread out all over the bed trying to figure out exactly where this trail goes, and where we'll stay the first couple nights on the trail.

So far, no luck finding any lodging for the first night of the South Leinster Way. I sent out two emails to places a few miles off the trail to see what might be available for lodging.

The day-to-day planning and mileage estimates for this next part of our hike, without a guidebook and detailed trail description, is going to be different, and a little more challenging.

Day #8
Boley Bridge and Central House B&B to Clonegal – 10 Miles
Total – 91.2 Miles

We got to the end of the Wicklow Way today. It's the most popular multi-day hiking trail in Ireland. Maybe tied with the Kerry Way that we'll get to in three weeks or so.

We ended up hiking about 10 more miles than the 81-mile length of the Wicklow Way. Mostly because we decided to start our hike at Temple Bar in downtown Dublin. That added about six miles just to get to the official start of the Wicklow. And then we added two miles by taking the Miner's Way alternate route the other day out of Glendalough. And we also walked about two extra miles around the lower lake at Glendalough the day before. So, our total at the official end of this first trail is a little over 91 miles by the end of today.

Completing the Wicklow Way is definitely an accomplishment. And it was fun! For most people who set a goal of through-hiking a trail in Ireland, they either hike the Wicklow Way or the Kerry Way. Since there is no designated cross-Ireland trail, no defined route, and no detailed hiking trail guides for the next three weeks, we're a little more on our own starting today. One trail down and four more to go.

It was pretty anticlimactic getting to the end of this first trail on our cross-Ireland hike. Partly because tomorrow morning we'll just wake up, put on our packs, and keep going. And partly because there is literally no sign post or marker that says that Clonegal is the end (or the beginning, depending on which way you are hiking) of the Wicklow Way.

Nothing.

Just a sign that points the direction of the trail heading back in the direction of Dublin and Marlay Park that looks exactly like the hundreds of trail signs that we've seen all along the way over the past eight days.

There was a fun part about finishing our hike as we walked into the village of Clonegal today. As we got to the end of the Wicklow Way, which consists of a little gazebo in a very small park, the four kids that we've been hiking with the last few days were standing there shivering in the rain.

They'd camped last night, somewhere beyond Boley Bridge and Shillellagh, where we'd stopped, and then got going early this morning. They'd been standing beneath the gazebo for three hours, waiting for Daniel and Niamh's dad to pick them up. None of them had a raincoat. Too much extra weight to carry for these lightweight backpackers. Everyone was noticeably shivering. It was great to bump into them one last time.

Really nice people.

We exchanged email addresses and Facebook info, and then Leslie and I headed off to call for a ride to our lodging for the night. We had a tough time finding a place to stay when I was calling around a few nights ago.

We called Phil our host at Meadowside B&B in Bunclody for a ride. Bunclody is six to seven miles south of Clonegal, and the closest place we could find to spend the night.

Today's hike went by pretty quickly. Breakfast at the Central House was sort of a do-it-yourself deal. But just fine. It was actually a nice break from eggs and ham and sausage.

We met a couple at dinner last night, sitting outside the Parkview House. Both in their 70s and very avid hikers. They had just started in Clonegal that morning, heading in the other direction. They were just carrying daypacks and having their luggage transported ahead each day, but still—early 70s!! Very impressive!!

They are members of some international hiking club, and go on hikes all over the world. They had participated in some kind of "officially sanctioned" thing, where you go on a specific designated day hike in each of the fifty U.S. states, and in all of the provinces in Canada, which they have done.

The guy was somewhat overweight (join the club), and walked kind of hunched over. Leslie and I were amazed at their plan to hike the entire Wicklow Way, and wondered, especially, whether the guy knew what he was getting into. The lady, also very nice, had a bit of a "peak bagger" mentality. For example, she said she'd only hiked the very last bit of the El Camino Trail in Spain so that she could "get the certificate."

I mailed off some stuff that I just haven't been using. Getting rid of my lightweight down jacket, two empty stuff sacks, an extra map case, and an unused phone power cord was more of a psychological boost than actually dropping much weight from my backpack. But why carry this stuff for another three to four weeks?

Phil, the owner of Central House, gave us a ride back to Boley Bridge around 9:30am, and it almost immediately started to rain. Our first real rain in eight days!!

The route started out heading straight uphill, and continued uphill for the first three miles along a very narrow one-lane country road that turned into a tractor path, and then a footpath. We had our backpack rain covers on all day. We took our raincoats on and off several times during the day as the rain started and stopped.

With about two miles to go in our relatively short hiking day today, it started raining pretty hard, and continued pouring all the way to Clonegal where we met the kids.

About a half-mile out of town, we passed two local walkers who were just out for their afternoon walk . . . in the pouring rain. One lady looked to be in her 50s and the other was a younger woman. Pouring rain. No raincoats. Just heavy knit wool sweaters. The older lady stopped to ask if we'd hiked all the way from Dublin, where we'd stayed; and what the trail was like along the way. She said she'd love to hike the Wicklow Way with her husband someday. I said, "Go for it. Don't wait. Do it while you can."

Meadowside B&B is owned by a wonderful older lady named Phil. She's had the B&B for over 30 years, and used to own the clothing boutique next door for over 40 years. Super nice.

She originally said she was full when I'd called a couple of days ago. But when I told her that we were hiking the Wicklow Way, she decided to rent us a room that has a bathroom down the hall, which was fine. Especially since there was nothing in Clonegal, and absolutely nothing in Bunclody.

We walked to Sorentino's for dinner, in the center of Bunclody. A cute little village. We actually headed out from the Meadowside going in the wrong direction, and walked about a half-mile before I realized the restaurant was in the other direction. Extra walking is such a bummer, especially since Leslie's feet have been throbbing all day long. We grabbed a few groceries at the SPAR on the way back, and now are all settled in for the night.

I forgot to mention our meeting with Simon yesterday. We were about halfway done with our hike to Boley Bridge, maybe less than that. It was late morning. We were walking down a trail and a middle-aged guy and his wife were coming uphill through a gate on the trail. Simon stopped to talk, and his wife just kept on walking.

Simon was super funny, and transitioned from talking about how Ireland's entry into the European Union had ruined the country to how the Catholic church had completely controlled the country and the minds of Irish people for centuries, until just a few decades ago; and from how Dublin is not really Ireland because most of the people living there these days are from somewhere else to what a drunken sod he used to be.

Simon told us a hilarious story about how he'd befriended a guy from Kenya (he wasn't actually sure what African country this guy was from), who had some kind of tribal scars on his cheeks. This guy had apparently invited Simon to a huge party somewhere in London, where he was living at the time. Simon ended up getting so drunk at the party that he woke up the next morning underneath a table.

Simon said that he doesn't drink anymore.

He said that he hates the idea of "drinking responsibly" because it's no fun. He either wants to drink a lot and get drunk, or not at all. So, he's chosen, "not at all."

Simon said that his brother is an alcoholic. "He's going to die soon. I don't want him to, because I like him. But I'm sure he'll be dead soon."

Simon threw a lot of "fockin' this" and "fockin' that" into every story, and reminded us several times of how the Catholic church controlled people's minds. Especially old people. He said Ireland is now only 10 percent Catholic, whereas a few decades ago it was 80 percent Catholic. This is all according to Simon, but we got his point.

On and on and on he went. Who knows where his wife was off to. But Leslie and I were really glad that we stopped to talk with Simon!

Day #9
Day #1 – South Leinster Way
Clonegal to Kildavin (Start of the South Leinster Way) to Chasell's
Cross and Brenda's B&B in Boris – 13.4 Miles
Total – 104.6 Miles

Leslie is an amazing, bad ass hiker!

When she got out of bed this morning, she could barely walk. The tops of her feet are super painful. No idea if it's muscles, or joints, or small stress fractures? But she could literally not put any pressure on them when walking around. She had to hold on to things to limp to the bathroom and while packing up this morning.

She spent a few minutes trying to stretch out her feet, loaded up on three Advil, and off we went.

The same taxi guy that Phil called yesterday afternoon picked us up at 9am and drove us back to the end of the Wicklow Way in Clonegal. Two German women, who were also staying at the Meadowside, rode with us to start their Wicklow Way hike heading back towards Dublin. They, and everyone else we've seen and met (other than the kids), are using a baggage service to haul their bags to their next stop. It makes us old people feel a little tougher. And also probably the reason for Leslie's tender feet.

The weather predictions for today changed several times, and mostly for the better. It was super windy all day, blowing 20 to 25 miles per hour, especially above the trees. It rained three different times during the day. Each time, we could see the rain coming towards us from off in the distance, so we had time to take off our packs and put on our raincoats and rain pants. And then, 15 to 20 minutes later, once the rain had passed, we'd take it all off again and just hike in a windbreaker.

Leslie has worn long pants for the last few days. I much prefer shorts. So, the wind and the rain made for a chilly day. But other than the rain, it was a perfect day for hiking.

Route Details for Day 1 on the South Leinster Way

Since there isn't a guidebook for the South Leinster Way, I'm adding some route details that I didn't include for the Wicklow Way section.

Clonegal (end of the Wicklow Way) to Kildavin (start of the South Leinster Way)—since these two trails don't actually connect, you need to walk about two and a half miles of road with no roadside up and over a few hills, so watch for traffic. There was very little traffic for a Saturday.

The South Leinster Way starts at a posted sign that is across the street from Conway's Bar in Kildavin. (There is no lodging in Kildavin, by the way. Bunclody as the nearest lodging to the start of this trail.) Walk a quarter of a mile to cross over busy N80, and then about a mile and a half mostly uphill to the end of a paved road.

Take a grassy path to the left. It is signed, but was totally overgrown and we missed it at first. It's a pretty stiff uphill hike through a forest to a grassy track. There is an overgrown sign that points to the right at this trail cross section. After that turn, the route is fairly well signed to the intersection with a paved road.

Go about three miles on a steep uphill, and then left to another long uphill that continues above the tree line and around Mount Leinster. This section is very exposed, especially when it's windy.

Go two and a half miles to "Nine Stones" and then downhill on a narrow tarmac road for just over three and a half miles to "Cashell's Cross" (a cross-roads about four to five kilometers before the small village of Boris). We stopped at Cashell's Cross and got a ride to our lodging in Boris.

Finding lodging at the end of our first day's walk on the South Leinster Way was difficult. It was a Saturday, and the first weekend of summer break for kids. There was also a big wedding in Boris that took up all the rooms in the one (expensive) lodging in Boris. And the fact of the matter is, out in this part of the country, there just aren't many lodging options. It's best to book several days in advance.

We finally got ahold of Connor and Brenda, at Brenda's B&B, south of Boris. Both absolutely wonderful people. I called Connor when we got to Cashell's Cross and he came and picked us up for a small fee.

If we hadn't started in Clonegal this morning, and instead had just started at the beginning of the South Leinster Way in Kildavin, we could have easily continued on into Boris for a 13-and-a-half-mile day, and not needed a ride. But the extra two and a half miles from Cashell's Cross was just more than we wanted to hike at the end of our day.

Walking and not getting a ride for that section that connected the end of the Wicklow Way to the start of the South Leinster Way was important to us. If you're going to through-hike something, like hiking across Ireland, than my ethic is that you hike every step, even when the trails don't connect. Other people might see it differently.

I remember when I through-paddled the Mississippi River a few years ago we met another paddler who said that he didn't think he needed to paddle across some of the huge lakes in Minnesota that the river passes through, Lake Winnibegosh and Lake Peppin, because they were lakes and not actually the river. He's the guy that said to us, "My trip. My rules."

The walk on the road from Clonegal to Kildavin this morning was along a quiet narrow lane that eventually crossed a river before reaching Kildavin. Leslie's feet were super painful and she walked with a bit of a limp. She's not complaining at all, but I know she's in pain, especially waiting for the Advil to kick in.

Around mile seven today, we broke out of the trees and onto a road, and saw that the road went straight uphill. The kind of steep hill that you have to get off your bike and walk up. We headed around a corner and rose above the tree line, and as the narrow road wound around the side of Mt. Leinster, we were hit with the full force of wind and driving rain. Above the trees, the road around the side of the mountain was super exposed.

It was a Saturday, and a fair number of cars passed us, probably wondering what the heck we were doing out in this weather. I was in a bit of a foul mood because the road just kept climbing, and the weather sucked.

We could see some cars parked at the top of the pass, a mile or two up ahead, and I kiddingly said, "Wouldn't it be great if there was a snack wagon (food truck) at the top, with hot cocoa?" The top of this pass was labeled "Nine Stones" on our map.

Well . . .

When we got to the top, there were dozens of cars and 70 or 80 people and a sign that read, "Poc Fada."

And . . . a snack wagon with coffee and hot cocoa, and a second one selling ice cream, which I thought was hilarious, since it was freezing cold and raining.

While waiting for my latte and Leslie's hot cocoa, the lady told me that "Poc Fada" means "long puck" which is a tournament for displaying various types of hurling skills, hurling being the national sport of Ireland—a sport that I've never seen and not sure I've even heard of.

In a Poc Fada tournament, each participant competes individually, using a wooden hurling stick, called a "hurley" (a long handled wooden stick with a wide flat paddle at one end), to smack a hurling ball, called a "sliotar" (pronounced "slither"), as far as they can. In this particular Poc Fada, the competitors had to keep hitting their sliotar as far as they could, along a two-kilometer route, which in this case was straight up a treeless mountain ridge with a constant 20 miles per hour wind that blew the small sliotar ball all over the place. So, smack it as far as you can, go to where the ball lands, and smack it again further along the route. The winner is the person who travels the two-kilometer course in as few hits as possible. That's "Long Puck" or Poc Fada.

I got most of this info from a guy who was there watching with his wife and his two small kids. We sat for a while at a picnic table on this mountain pass, watching and resting and trying to stay warm in the cold biting wind.

It wasn't until I did some Googling this evening that we learned that the "Nine Stones" were a series of several two-foot high ancient stones that were partly buried in the hillside. Depending on the legend you believe, the nine stones either commemorate nine local chieftains from centuries ago, or nine shepherds from long ago, or nine rebels who were killed in 1798.

The rest of our hike today was downhill, and included one short but very heavy rain shower shortly after we started off after our rest stop at Poc Fada. The rain storm once again involved stopping to put our rain gear back on, and then taking it all back off a short while later.

Beautiful scenery through stunning countryside. We also walked past some really old abandoned stone buildings. This area just feels like people have inhabited it for millennia.

When we got to Chasel Cross, a rural crossroad with not a single sign that said anything about Chasel, or a cross, I called Brenda's B&B. Brenda's husband Connor set out to get us. There was a very old stone farmhouse across the street from where we waited for our ride, and as we sat on a ancient stone wall, Spike the farm dog came over and jumped on Leslie for a good petting.

A few minutes later, Marty, the 78-year-old farmer who lived at Chasel Cross, came over to see who the heck we were.

I told Marty, "We're waiting for a ride from Brenda's B&B. Do you think he'll find us? I had a hard time giving him directions."

"You're a big enough guy. I think he'll see you."

"Are you saying I'm fat?" I asked as I patted my oversized belly.

"No. No. You're just a tall guy. If you were 22 years old, I'd hire you to help me haul silage for my cows."

As Connor's car pulled up, Marty said, "Oh, you should've told me it was this guy. He used to be my banker, and I owe him money."

We settled into Brenda's. She had some kind of illness that had taken her out of commission, so Connor showed us to our room and told us about breakfast. We could tell that he wasn't usually the one who met the guests. After a quick shower, Connor agreed to give us a ride into Boris so we could get some dinner. Downtown was only a mile away, but neither of us felt much like doing any more walking.

We got lamb kabobs at Benny's Takeout, and then walked across the street to Joyce's Pub for Guinness and to eat our kabobs. There were lots of locals in the pub watching a big soccer match. The beer tasted great, and the kabobs were gigantic and messy.

John, the bartender, met us at the door and asked if we were on holiday. He couldn't believe that we'd walked from Dublin and were continuing on tomorrow.

He kept saying, "Fucking hell."
"How many days will it take you to get to Valentia Island?" he asked.

"Around 30 to 32 days,"

"Fucking hell."

Earlier, when Connor picked us up at Chasel Cross, he was listening to his County Claire soccer team playing in Dublin at a national soccer tournament. When he drove us into Boris for dinner, he seemed crestfallen, so I asked, "How did County Claire do?" He frowned and said, "Good thing I took my heart pill."

Soccer is huge here, and the county teams are like our NFL teams. And team loyalty is fierce and in evidence everywhere. Connor had a County Claire banner flying in his front yard.

Connor told us to ask at Joyce's for a taxi home. He had a meeting and couldn't pick us up. When we were ready to head home, John the bartender, said, "Oh, I'd run you back but the bar is too busy." So, he got another regular to take us home. Paddy. Who appeared to have been drinking for quite a while. So, we piled in Paddy's car and he carefully and drunkenly drove us the mile back to Brenda's.

Only in Ireland.

Day #10
Day #2 – South Leinster Way
Chasell's Cross in Boris to Graiguenamanagh – 11 Miles
Total – 115.6 Miles

Route Details for Day 2 on the South Leinster Way

We walked three and a quarter miles from Chasel Cross along narrow country roads that were well signed. The "trail" leads right through downtown Boris for about one mile. Then left for three-quarters of a mile down to the Barrow River Bridge, and then left again along the left side of the river. We followed the river on a grassy dirt path for six miles past several small wooden locks. Seeing Graiguenamanagh approaching on the right side of the river, we eventually crossed a road bridge into town. The entire route was well signed.

It was a beautiful walking day.

Leslie's feet are still really painful. She's taped them up to pull her arches up (a trick she's used on previous long-distance hikes). It seemed to help a little. But the first few and last few miles of the day, she limps noticeably. My feet and legs and joints start aching usually around mile seven or eight. Hiking without packs would make a big difference, along with being 30 or 40 years younger!

We're staying at a really cute old inn, the Waterside Inn in Graiguenamanagh. Right on the River Barrow. There are dozens and dozens of old houseboats lining both sides of the river. It has the feel of a seaside village, even though we are around 50 miles from the ocean. The boats and the water make it feel like we're walking along the coast of Wales or England.

The weather forecast for today was originally for 80 to 100 percent chance of rain all day long. So, we were mentally ready to hike in the rain, but by the time we woke up this morning, the forecast had changed to scattered showers throughout the day, which is what we had. We walked through five or six little rain storms, one every hour or so.

The pub last night in Chasel Cross, where we ate our kabobs, was constructed of old stone walls and low ceilings. It was full of people, many from a local wedding, and the rest were watching the national soccer matches on TV.

Leslie and I each drank a pint and a half of Guinness while we ate our massive lamb kabobs (that were delicious), and more than we could finish. I also bought six small chicken wings, apparently because I'm always worried about not having enough food. I ended up eating the unrefrigerated wings on our rainy hike today.

After getting a ride back to where we stopped yesterday, our first three and a quarter miles traveled along narrow country roads that headed from Chasel Cross into Boris, then uphill through the long strung out town of Boris and past Benny's and Joyce's where we ate and drank last night. We stopped at a picnic table that sits in front of Joyce's for a rest and so Leslie could re-tape her aching feet.

Another almost two miles of road walking got us to the grassy path that runs along the River Barrow. It's actually a man-made canal, complete with several small working locks. It reminded me of our three-week bicycle trip along the Eric Canal in Upstate New York back in 2021.

After 13 or 14 miles of road walking yesterday and this morning, it was nice to be on a dirt and grass path. Other than a couple of joggers, we didn't see anyone on the trail. We did walk past three small camping tents that were set up alongside the path, and we heard voices coming out of them as we walked past around 1pm. Not sure what they were doing. They may have been hikers who stopped to avoid the rain?

We passed a small public swimming area, complete with two life-guard stands along the canal shore, which seemed kind of weird to me. At one point, as we neared Graig, a group of 10 river kayaks paddled past us and headed up the canal.

Despite the change in scenery and the pleasant flat walking, it was sort of a boring hiking day. Leslie carefully rationed her Advil throughout the day, not wanting to ingest her daily limit too early in the day.

We never got the hard, consistent rain that we expected. Just five or six fairly short showers, with a little intermittent sunshine thrown in.

Graiguenamanagh is a cool old village with lots of history, including 480-year-old stone bridges over the River Barrow, a small castle built in 1620, a stone animal pound built in the early 1800s to hold livestock seized from people who were compelled to give tithes to the local Catholic church, and a Cistercian Abbey that was built in the 1200s. Lots of stuff that we won't be exploring because by the end of the day, all we want to do is eat and lay in bed . . . too tired and achy to outweigh my curiosity.

Dinner tonight was a bust. We were hoping for Chinese food. Just something different that we could find in a slightly larger town, but they only had takeout, which we didn't feel like since it was still raining on and off.

We ended up in the Globe Pub, eating burgers, creamy vegetable soup, and nachos. All very disappointing.

Leslie has been pointing out that every single pub we've been in so far that serves food has had creamy vegetable soup as the Soup of the Day. Weird.

Day #11
Day #3 – South Leinster Way
Graiguenamanagh to Inistioge – 11.5 Miles
Total – 127.1 Miles

Route Details for Day 3 on the South Leinster Way

Head from River Barrow through town, across a busy road (R705); take the first left onto a narrow country lane (unsigned) and go uphill past Brandon Hill Glamping about two miles to where the asphalt road ends, and a forest track begins. All well signed.

Continue uphill along the trail that heads to the summit of Brandon Hill, but stay on the South Leinster Way to circle around Brandon Hill rather than taking the trail to the top. Most of the next six miles is in the forest, but there are some rewarding panoramic views along the way.

Continue through the forest to a narrow country lane that heads downhill for two and a half miles to a bridge over River Nore, and into Instioge.

We're all settled into our room at the Woodstock Inn in Instioge. Annette and Richard are the owners, and both were super friendly and welcoming. We love walking into a town and straight to lodging that is right off the trail. In this case, we're staying just a block away from the signed South Leister Way. And when there is food at the place we're staying, it's an extra bonus, since neither of us wants to walk anywhere after we've already been walking for most of the day.

While we were having dinner in the outdoor seating at the Woodstock, Annette came out and introduced herself and immediately offered to do our laundry!! We've been wishing for someone like Annette to offer up the opportunity to wash our clothes for the past several days. But, I'd asked the owner of the Waterside Inn in Graig yesterday afternoon if they could do a load of laundry, and he agreed. So, we actually are carrying all clean clothes and didn't take Annette up on her kind offer.

But back to this morning. Breakfast at the Waterside was the best yet. Lots of choices. Leslie got porridge and fresh fruit, and I got a pancake/crêpe and fruit. Both were delicious.

Today's hike was pretty non-descript.

A few lame highlights:

1. We stopped at a pharmacy on our way out of Graig, and Leslie bought a hairbrush, Tylenol, and more medical tape to wrap her feet. She is walking in pain all day long, but remembered this morning, that on our two-month Wales Coast Path hike, a combo of Advil and Tylenol seemed to help.

2. We lost the "trail" heading out of Graig. At a turn, about three-quarters of a mile out of town, there was no trail sign so we kept walking straight along a country lane. Maybe 400 yards past where we were supposed to turn, I started thinking we'd made a mistake. As I was standing literally in the middle of the country road we were on, with my map open, a local guy stopped his truck to offer his help, confirming that we'd missed the turnoff. He offered to give us a ride back to the turn, and then up the hill to where the trail heads into the woods (about two miles). But we declined. Actually, the owner of the Waterside Inn offered to drive us to the same spot earlier this morning. We explained that we are walking across Ireland. Not walking and getting rides. A detail that seems lost on most people we try to explain it to.

3. The walk was mostly through the forest on a dirt, rock, and gravel track. Boring, but it went by pretty quickly. We both felt a lot better physically today. Better than yesterday. I actually cranked up the hills ahead of Leslie today. Of course, she's been totally hobbling, limping, and in pain . . . but still. . . .

4. The flies were really bad for several miles in the woods. No breeze. Literally hundreds of swarming flies buzzing around our heads, in my ears, and in my eyes at any given moment. I think Leslie swallowed a couple. So obnoxious! They don't bite, but just the feeling of them in my hair and walking across my face drove me crazy!! They don't seem to swarm around Leslie's head as much as mine. She keeps saying it's because I don't put on deodorant. Which is factually true. But I don't think the flies know.

Leslie's new drug cocktail seemed to really help. Along with her frequent foot stretches, and foot massages when we stop for breaks, and when she takes off her shoes. This evening she just said that her feet feel better than they have in days!!

After dinner tonight, I talked with Richard at the bar in the pub downstairs from our room. We talked about Irish whiskey. Richard said that a good Irish whiskey is far superior to a good single malt Scotch. He said that Scotch gets all the headlines, especially in the States, but that good Irish whiskey is much better and significantly less expensive. Richard showed me a bottle of 12-year-old Irish whiskey that smelled super peaty, and he said that a similar bottle of Scotch would cost four times the price. There are definitely plenty of pubs up ahead where I can put his theory to the test.

Richard also told me that Irish people don't just sip whiskey straight, either neat or over ice. They always mix it with either water or soda. He also introduced me to several brands of "working man's whiskey," which basically meant that they were all affordable for the average person. So, one of these evenings, when we don't have very far to hike the next day, I'm going to try some Irish whiskey.

Tomorrow looks like a longer day, a good 14 miles or more to get to the place we reserved in Mullinavat. Apparently the 2022 Irish Open (golf) is this weekend at a private course that is only about five miles from here. We've been warned that lodging could be a problem these next few days.

Day #12
Day #4 – South Leinster Way
Inistioge to Mullinavat (Garrandarragh Inn at Rising Star) – 13.4 Miles
Total – 140.5 Miles

We're both happy that today is over with.

Route Details for Day 4 on the South Leinster Way

The initial three-quarters of a mile out of Instioge is along the river. Then hike two and a half miles uphill through trees to cross a tarmac road. Follow a forest track for about six miles that travels through dense forest and some clear-cut open areas. Then follow country roads for the remaining five miles into Mullinavat.

We'd been checking the weather frequently over the past 24 hours. Watching the weather on my numerous weather, wind, and satellite apps is part of my morning, afternoon, and evening ritual. Today's weather pretty much matched the forecasts.

We woke to hard driving rain at 6am. With the wind blowing 20 to 25 miles per hour. The trees outside our window were bending over. It was nasty. A total hiker buzzkill.

We dawdled around a bit after our 8am breakfast, delaying the inevitable. But when we finally walked out the door at 9:15am, the rain was blowing almost sideways, and it stayed that way for the next two hours.

We were both wearing lightweight, single-membrane raincoats and rain pants, so they weren't made from some kind of breathable Gore-Tex. Consequently, with lots of exertion, condensation builds up on the inside of our rain shells, and the inside ends up as wet as the outside. At some point, our outerwear really just helps to cut the wind and keep body heat in.

So, it was just a cold, wet, and windy first two hours of walking. We were both soaked to the skin. The key is to just keep moving so you don't get chilled. It was the kind of driving rain that just runs down your face. Like standing in a cold shower.

We walked through two or three more brief showers during the day. Enough to keep our pack covers on, and our raincoats close by.

The wind blew all day long, which helped dry us out between showers.

Just a long cold, wet walk.

We stopped for a brief lunch around mile seven—peanut butter on crackers, a raisin and nut concoction that we'd thrown together,protein bars. Nothing to look forward to. Just fuel to stay warm and keep hiking.

Leslie was back to significantly limping for most of the way today. Her Tylenol and Advil cocktail never really seemed to kick in. It was hard to watch, and I know she was in a lot of pain.

There is nothing in Mullinavat except the Garrandaragh Inn, a Centra Mini Mart, a fast food takeout place, and the Enchanted Garden Thai restaurant. We'd heard about the Thai restaurant from William, who owned the Woodstock. William said that the owners were from Thailand. We'd even checked the menu online a couple of times and knew what we were going to order hours before we got to Mullinavat. Such are the food obsessions of a mind with not much else to think about.

Our plan was to order takeout and eat in our room while watching the fifth "episode" of the January 6, 2021, U.S. Capitol insurrection hearings being held by the House of Representatives, which focused on the storming of the Capitol by armed thugs and Trump supporters.

Calling the Enchanted Garden and finding out that they were closed on Tuesdays was devastating.

I spent the evening catching up on work, phone calls, and watching the hearings.

We're planning a short day tomorrow to give Leslie's feet a chance to heal a little. And then I'm planning our hike and lodging so that we can walk for part of Thursday and all day Friday without our packs, hoping that will help Leslie's feet as well.

And I think that Carrick-on-Suir, where we'll be tomorrow night, is a big enough town to have sporting goods stores that sell supportive shoe insoles. Even the bottoms of my feet were aching after so much road walking today.

Just not a fun day.

But that's all part of the deal. Part of the adventure.

If it was easy, everyone would be hiking across Ireland.

Not really.

About a mile and a half before we got to Mullinavat this afternoon, we were plodding along the shoulder of a paved road when an old guy came out of his house and called me over. He asked if we needed any water, and then if we wanted to come in for tea or coffee.

So nice.

If it had been earlier in the day, or still raining, we'd have gone in in a second. But we only had a mile and a half to go, and we both just wanted to be done for the day.

Looking back, I regret not taking him up on his offer for tea.

Day #13
Day #5 – South Leinster Way
Mullinavat to Pilstown (taxi to Carrick-on-Suir) – 9 Miles
Total – 149.5 Miles

Route Details for Day 5 on the South Leinster Way

One hundred percent road walking. We only went nine miles today, walking over rolling hills. Nothing steep or sustained. Great views of farmland and distant mountains. Easy walking. Very peaceful.

"A dog at the end of every driveway."

We are sitting in Comeragh Pub, having a pint before we find dinner here in Carrick-on-Suir. Chatting it up with the lady bartender and another lady who is sitting at the bar and having a drink.

I went up to the bar to ask them if they'd judge today's photo contest.

Earlier today, Leslie was getting really bored with our hike, and she said, "We haven't even played the 'what color car is coming up behind us' game or the 'how much do you think our meal will cost' game."

Me: "It's because we aren't bored enough yet."

Leslie: "I am."

So, she created the photo contest game.

Today's topic (picked by me) was "stone structures."

The rules are that we each take photos throughout the day of various things made out of stone (walls, buildings, old stone fences, or just randomly stacked stones). And at the end of the day, we'll find someone to judge our photos to see who won.

So, while sitting here at the Comeragh Pub, we each picked our best stone structure photo, and I showed them to the lady sitting at the bar.

She picked mine. Yes!

Jon - 1; Leslie - 0. Leslie will pick the topic of our photo contest tomorrow.

The other highlight of the day,was meeting Emma. We were walking along a narrow, windy country road towards the end of our short nine-mile hike today, and it looked like rain was heading our way. We stopped along the side of the road, took our packs off, and fished out our raincoats.

A woman in a long winter coat came down her driveway and introduced herself. Emma asked all about our hike, and couldn't believe that we'd walked all the way from Dublin. She said that she and her husband had just returned home after spending the weekend in Graiguenamanagh. She said that she was a walker, and someday she'd love to hike the Wicklow Way. But her husband is a farmer, and apparently not super healthy. Leslie encouraged Emma to find some girlfriends and do a girl's hike of the Wicklow Way.

We told Emma about Leslie's feet troubles, and she offered to drive us to our hotel tonight in Carrick-on-Suir. I'd mentioned that we are doing a shorter hike today only to Pilstown, and were planning to call a taxi to go the last five miles to our hotel. And then we'll return in the morning to walk that final five miles of the South Leinster Way.

I misunderstood Emma, and thought she'd offered to meet us in Pilstown and drive us to our hotel, so I said, "Sure, that'd be great. We should be there in 45 minutes if you want to pick us up then." Emma agreed to meet us in 45 minutes, and said it would be her "good deed for the day." It wasn't until we were walking away, that Leslie said, "That was really awkward. She wasn't offering to meet us in 45 minutes. She was offering to take us right now."

Ooops.

I felt a little embarrassed, but said, "People like to be helpful, and feel like they are helping us on our trip."

Emma did pick us up about two miles down the road, and drove us the five miles to the Cariegh Hotel. She also pointed out a couple of places where we could look for better insoles for Leslie's shoes. Emma asked us about our kids and grandkids. She has four adult children. One who just returned from living in Australia for the past three years. She has a daughter who lives in town. Her youngest is a 20-year-old boy who just got back yesterday from a trip to

Spain with his buddies. And then, Emma told us about her fourth, a 28-year-old boy who died tragically last year.

Emma said, "You have to live your life now. It's hard to live a balanced life, but we all need to find balance in our lives, and not focus too much on work." Seeming to question herself a little, she continued, "I think that's right, isn't it?"

Yes it is, Emma.

Leslie's feet were pretty bad again today. It was the reason we decided to hike only nine miles today. I'm worried that this will only get worse. She literally limps with every step.

New strategies for foot care include more foot massaging every morning and evening, icing them as soon as we get to the hotel (which we did), buy new, more supportive insoles (which we did), alter Tylenol/Advil cocktail a bit.

So, hopefully. . . .

Today we road walked the whole day. Five miles tomorrow morning and we'll walk into Carrick-on-Suir and the end of the South Leinster Way. I'm not 100 percent sure where the East Munster Way starts, but it's somewhere in Carrick-on-Suir.

We'll find it.

Day #14
Day #6 – South Leinster Way
Day #1 – East Munster Way
Pilstown through Carrick-on-Suir to Kilsheelan –12 Miles
Total – 161.5 Miles

Route Details

Five miles of rural road walking from Pilstown to Carrick-on-Suir and the end of the South Leinster Way. The start of the East Munster Way begins in the center of Carrick-on-Suir and heads seven miles along the Suir River (also known as Blue Way) to Kilsheelan.

It's already 9pm and I'm just getting around to writing.

We weren't able to get a taxi this morning back to Pilstown, where we left off yesterday, to finish the final five miles of the South Leinster Way. The two or three we called were all busy until 10am, probably doing school runs. I remember learning in England that lots of taxis have scheduled morning runs for kids who aren't on a school busline. So, we decided to walk the five miles "backwards" from Carrick-on-Suir back to Pilstown, and then taxi back the five miles so that we could continue our hike and begin the East Munster Way.

It's a funny thing about most through-hikers of long-distance trails. It doesn't matter which direction you go, or how you string the segments together, as long as you hike the entire route in a single effort. Even the idea of skipping a mile, or getting a ride for a short distance on the route, is against our self-imposed rules of through-hiking. No one else knows. No one else cares. But we do.

After walking back to Pilstown, we caught a taxi from Anthony's Pub. The taxi driver dropped us back at the Carraigh Hotel. I grabbed my half-empty backpack of things we'd need for today's remaining seven miles, and then we sent the taxi on to our planned lodging in Clonmel with the rest of our stuff. Forcing ourselves to hike every step of the way with full backpacks is not one of our self-imposed rules of through-hiking.

We'd decided when we got up this morning that the best thing for Leslie's feet today would be to hire a taxi to bring our bags to the next town, and only hike with one daypack that I would carry. It's what just about everyone else we've met does every day of their through-hikes of the Wicklow Way, and even other long-distance hikes in the U.K. and Ireland. There are baggage transfer companies that just pick up your bags each morning and drive them to your next stop.

We've never done that. Maybe because it costs money, but also because it feels weird. Almost like we are cheating. Another self-imposed long-distance hiking ethic.

Walking all day without a pack seemed to helped Leslie's feet. And my pack of food, water, maps, first aid kit, and our rain gear was only 10 to 12 pounds.

Once Leslie's Advil and Tylenol kicked in, she moved pretty well. But once everything wears off, she's in a lot of pain.

Our first five miles went by quickly. With all of the rain these last few days, there was one spot where the country road that the route followed was under a couple feet of water. Thankfully there was an alternate path with a walking bridge, probably built for rainy periods like these.

The initial seven miles of the East Munster Way heading out of Carrick-on-Suir were beautiful and peaceful as the paved trail followed right along the north bank of the Suir River.

The photo contest today was, "Living things along the river that aren't people" (animals not plants). So, that kept us occupied. For the first few miles along the river, we saw absolutely no birds, ducks, or any sign of animal life. Instead, we both competed to take creative shots of bumble bees perched on flowers—what Leslie calls "sweat bees"—and flies. Super lame.

We eventually started seeing horses, cows, and some ducks floating on the river. We didn't have anyone to judge our photos tonight. We'll have to find someone over breakfast. My best one was of two bees sitting on the same bright yellow dandelion. Leslie's was a great one of some horses in a meadow. I think she's going to win.

Seven more miles got us to Kilsheelan, known as the "Tidiest Villages in Ireland." I think that means "cute."

We went to Nagles Pub and Restaurant. We originally wanted to spend the night in Nagles, but they were booked because of the Irish Open, and they were the only lodging in town. So we ended our day at the pub, and sat outside to enjoy a pint of cold Angry Orchard hard cider, and then got a taxi to Clonmel to meet up with our bags at Mulcahy's where we'll be for the next two nights.

Tomorrow, we'll taxi back to Nagles and then walk the 10 to 11 miles along the Munster Way to Clonmel.

We both spent a couple of hours trying to figure our lodging out for the next few days. The Munster Way heads out of Clonmel, and for the next 25 to 30 miles doesn't really go near any towns or villages or lodging. After lots of Googling, I don't have anything booked for the day after tomorrow or beyond because there isn't anything anywhere near the trail, and very few road crossings where we could try to catch a ride. This is the downside of not carrying a tent and sleeping bags on this trip.

We had dinner in Clonmel at an Asian street food place called

"Lana." Mostly Thai food on the menu, and it was really good! A great change from pub food.

Today was our 14th day of hiking. Not quite halfway. I think we are both in a bit of a lull in terms of hiking enthusiasm. Lots of paved road and paved paths the last few days. Tomorrow we head back up into the hills. But since we're just walking right into Clonmel, we'll only have my daypack again, so that'll be awesome. Hopefully Leslie's feet appreciate the break.

Day #15
Day #2 – East Munster Way
Kilsheelan to Clonmel – 8 Miles
Total – 169.5 Miles

I read an article in the news today about a guy who just completed his walk around the entire world!

He'd been walking for seven years, and walked 29,800 miles!!

He's the 10th person on record to walk around the world.

Apparently, there are rules about these things. You have to have crossed at least four continents and traveled a minimum of a certain number of miles to qualify as a legitimate around-the-world hiker.

There are rules and records for all kinds of adventures.

This guy said that it had been an obsession of his for the past 15 years, and that he was happy to be done. He currently has no interest in going anywhere. He just wants to stay at home for a while. He picked up a dog along the way. And a girlfriend.

We, on the other side of the walking spectrum, only hiked eight miles today. We'd set out to hike 12 and a half, from Kilsheelan up into the hills and then back down across the Suir and into Clonmel. But about three miles into our hike this morning, the marked East Munster Way went a different way than the map that I'd printed off the Internet showed. And the signed trail ended up cutting off over four miles. We were happy, since it rained for the final two miles. A misty, drizzly, soaking rain.

Along the way, we passed a small white country cottage, and Leslie said something about what a cute little cottage it was. As we passed, a lady came out the cottage door and jumped in her car. She proceeded to stop in the middle of the narrow lane, as she was passing us, to say hello. She told us that there was a "castle estate" across the street from her cottage, that ran along the River Suir. The owner of the estate owns all of the surrounding land, including the cute little cottage that she rents. She asked about our hike and was super encouraging. She's English, but moved from London to rural Clonmel "for a better quality of life."

Several cars came up behind her as we talked. Every time, I'd say, "Oh, we need to get out of the middle of the road." And every time, she'd reply, "Oh, they're fine. They can go around."

The East Munster Way left the road and wound up into the trees on a wooded track. We climbed for about a mile and a half, and then the trail departed from the mapped route. The route stayed in the trees, high up near the ridgeline, with some occasional great views of the river valley below. We could see the massive Bulmer's cider plant down below, a few miles away.

The last two and a half miles dropped back down along the River Suir, like much of yesterday's hike. We walked in the rain with our pack covers on. For some reason, I decided not to put my raincoat on, sure that the rain shower would only last a few minutes. So, after I was completely soaked to the skin, Leslie, who'd had her raincoat on the entire time, convinced me to put mine on too, since it was windy and cold. Too little, too late.

Because of our shortened hike today, we were back in our hotel in Clonmel by 1pm!

We called the same taxi driver who picked us up at the end of yesterday to get us to the start of our walk this morning. J.P. was very talkative, and for our ten-minute ride this morning he asked a lot of questions about our trip. J.P. was very clear about his belief that Donald Trump and his relationship with Putin could've averted Russia's attack and destruction of Ukraine.

Leslie and I made it clear that we couldn't stand Trump. I told J.P. that Putin had been playing Trump's ego (as in manipulating) for years.

J.P. also told us about Ronald Reagan's ancestors who lived nearby in Ballyporeen, a small village that we'll walk through tomorrow, and where J.P. is also from. He said that Reagan came to visit there when he was running for his second term in office to secure the Irish vote in the U.S.

J.P. also told us that Obama came to visit his ancestral land in Ireland, Ballygurteen, also in County Tipperary and also very nearby.

J.P. had a very funny way of talking. He'd say, "Well, lads. It's a sunny day today, isn't it, lads? So, where will you be walking today, lads?" He literally added "lads" to the end of every sentence . . . lads.

After our nap, I walked to a cute coffee place a couple of blocks down the street called The Hub. We had breakfast there this morning. Great coffee. I brought my laptop to get some work done, and Leslie took her time taking a shower and beautifying.

It actually felt weird being apart for a little over an hour. The first time in over two weeks. It was a funny feeling. I felt like something was missing.

J.P. told us that there were three pubs in Clonmel that were must-sees. One was the place where we were staying, Mulcahy's, the second was a tiny non-descript pub painted in black and a few blocks down the street from or hotel called Phil Carroll's Bar, and the third was the place where we decided to have dinner tonight, a pub painted bright red and across the street from The Hub called Sean Tierney's.

Sean Tierney's was a classic and well-known old Irish pub. It is known for the thousands of little knick-knacks that cover every square inch of the walls and shelves inside. J.P. told us that it was like a museum and he was right. Leslie ordered an Irish whiskey with ginger ale, that she loved, and I got a pint.

Unfortunately, dinner at Sean Tierney's was super disappointing. I got wings and mash with a salad. The wings were coated in dry spices, like the old Shake 'n Bake we had when we were kids. And the "salad" was just a tablespoon of coleslaw. Leslie ordered grilled salmon that was supposed to be poached, and was super dried out and fishy tasting. According to the Internet, Sean Tierney's is known for their good food, so I'm not sure what happened. It was so bad that I wrote a review on Tripadvisor (it's rare for me to write a review).

Overall, Clonmel is a cut town, with lots going on. J.P. told us it was the largest inland city in Ireland.

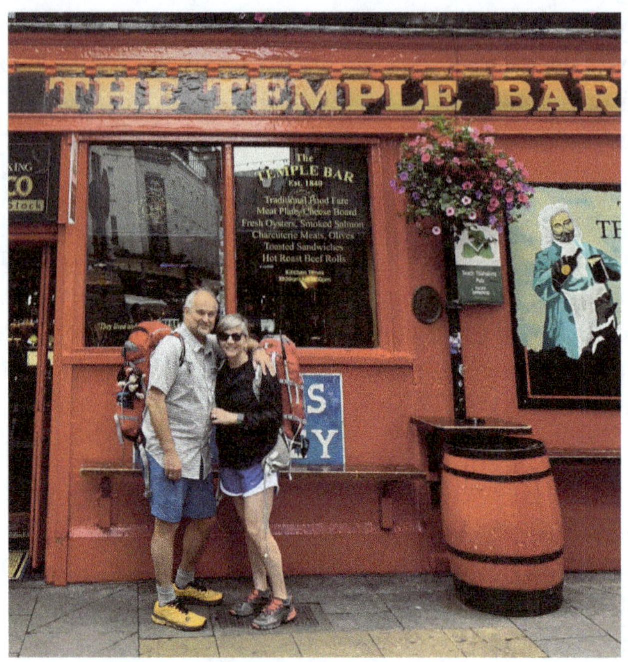

Temple Bar Pub, the start of our cross-Ireland hike

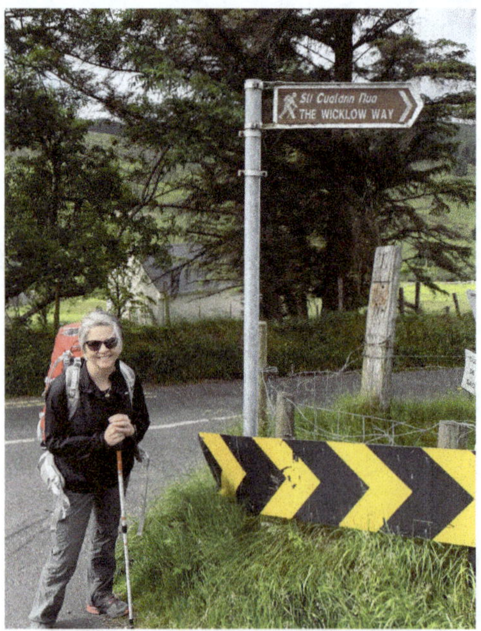

Day 1 on the Wicklow Way

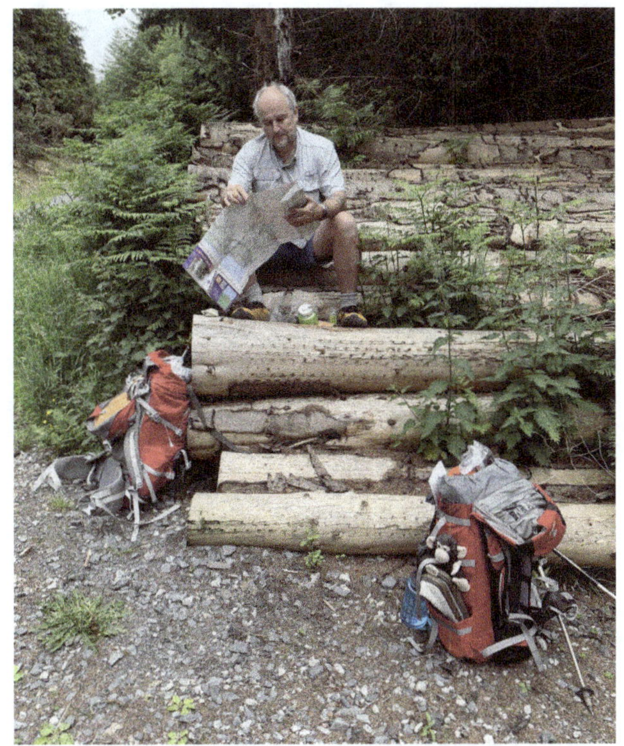

Checking the map

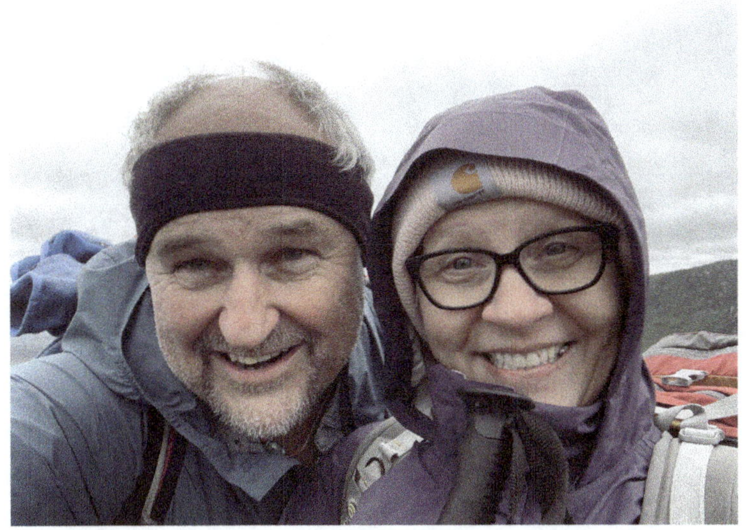

Cold and rainy in the Wicklow Mountains, Day 3

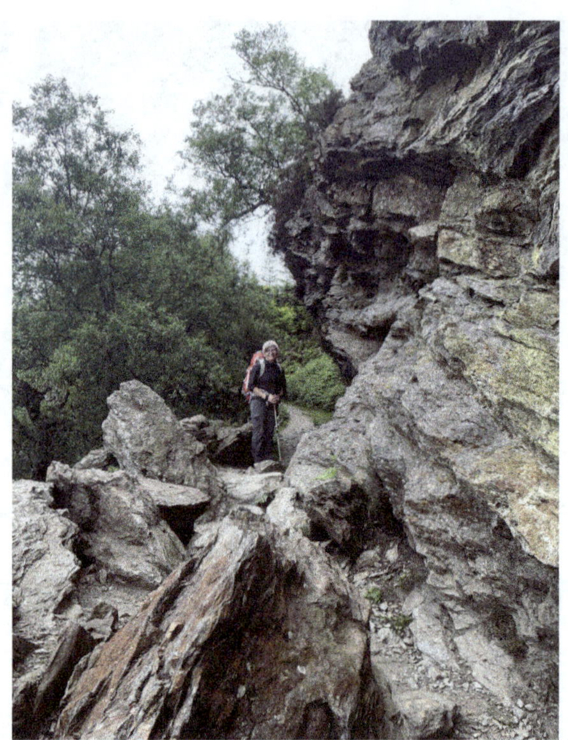

Approaching Powerscourt Waterfall,
Ireland's highest waterfall, Day 3

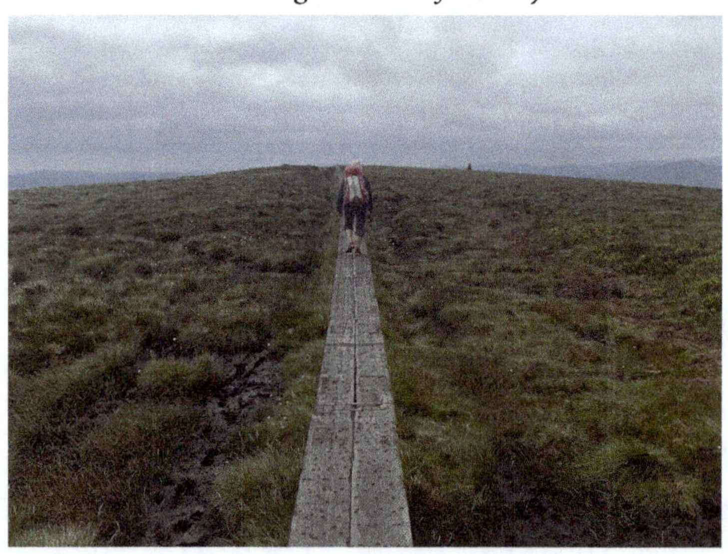

Hiking through the Wicklows

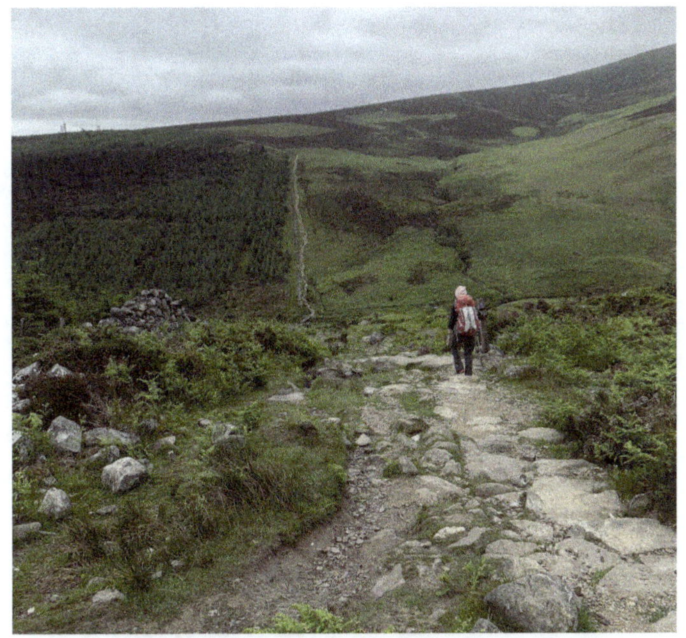

The Beautiful Wicklow Mountains

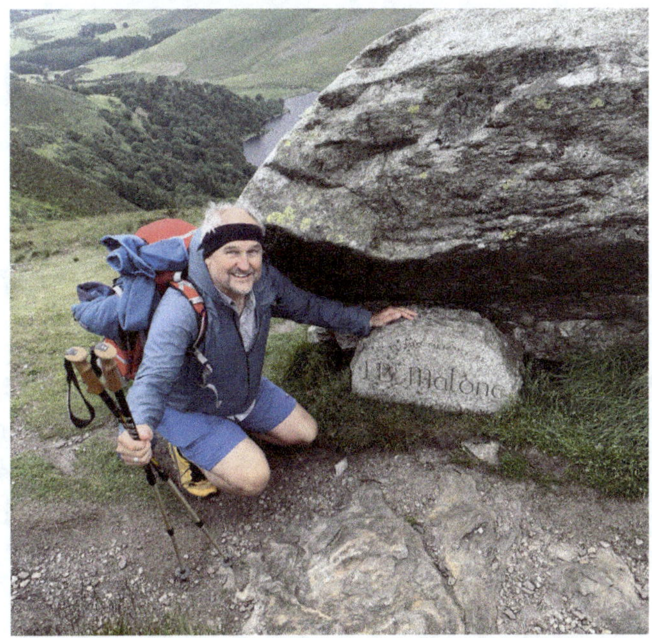

Memorial to J.B. Malone, responsible for establishing the Wicklow Way

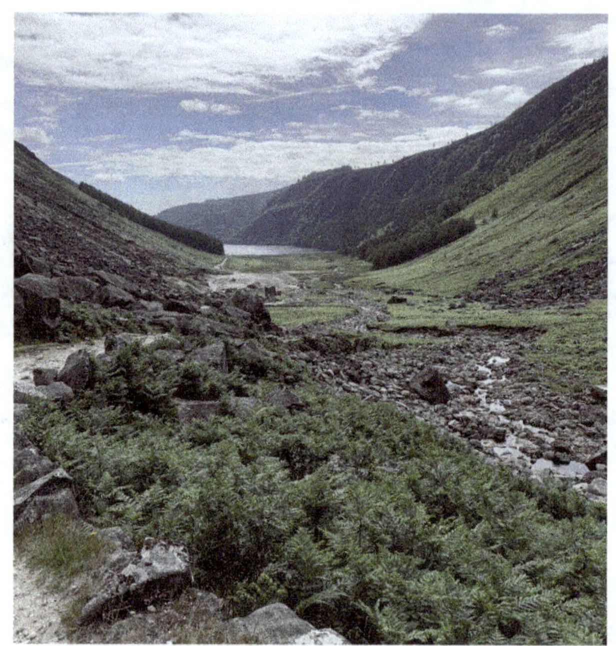

Van Diemen's Land above Upper Glendalough Lake

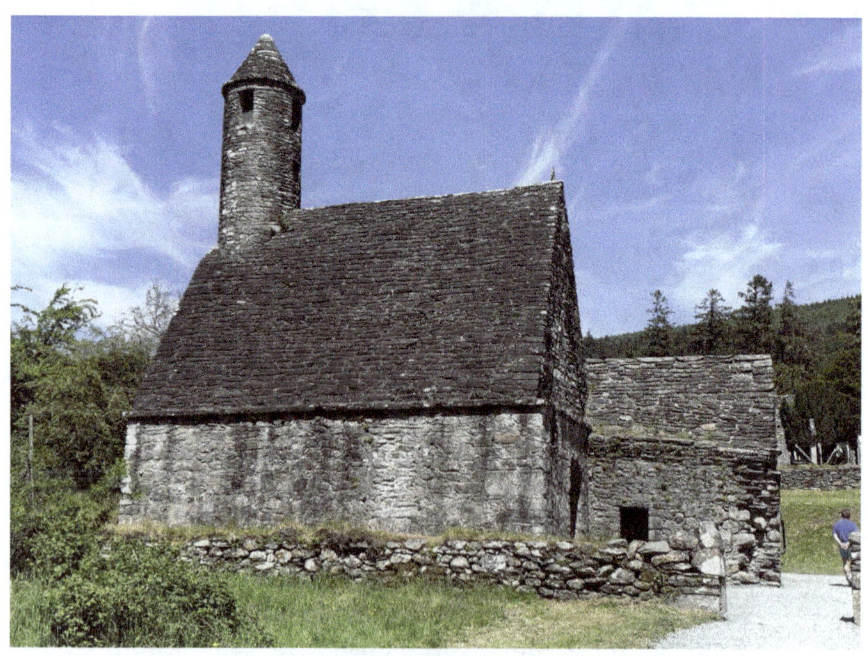

Stone church in Glendalough, Day 4

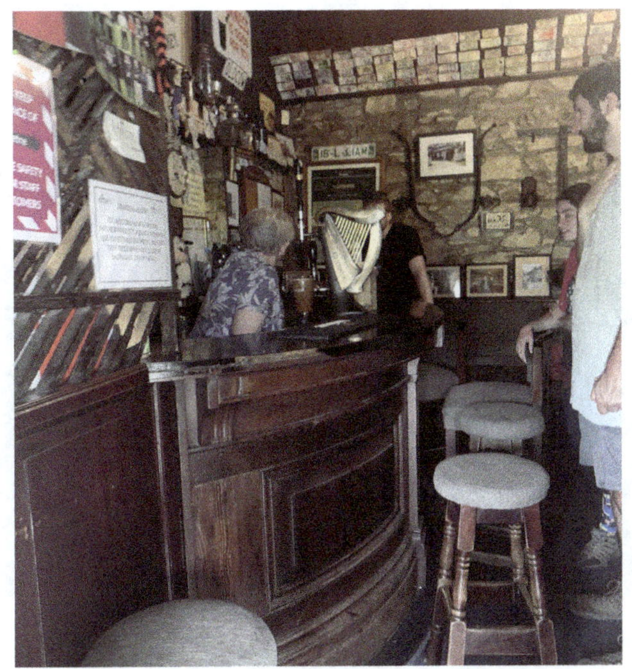

The Dying Cow (Tallon's) Pub, Day 7

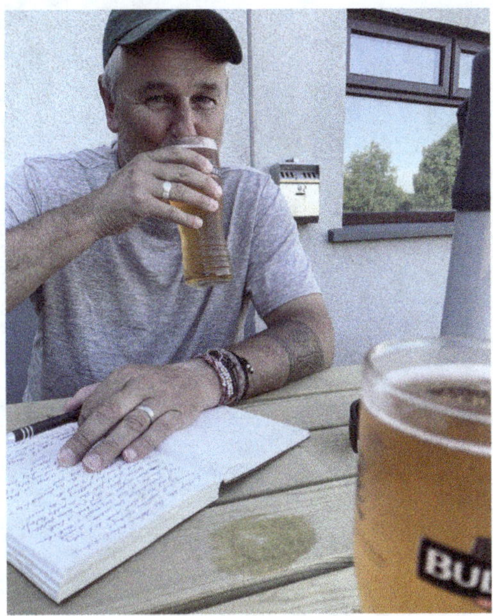

Two of my favorite parts of long-distance hiking

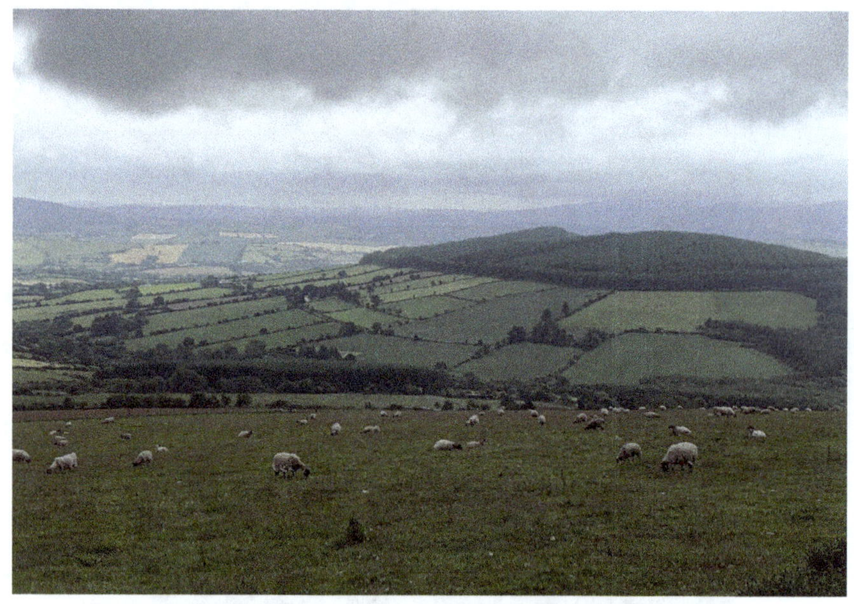

Walking to Clonegal, Day 8

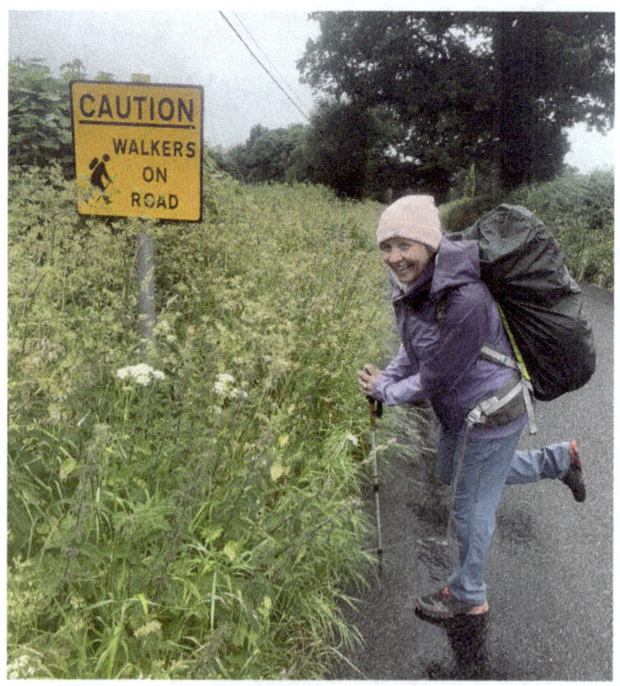

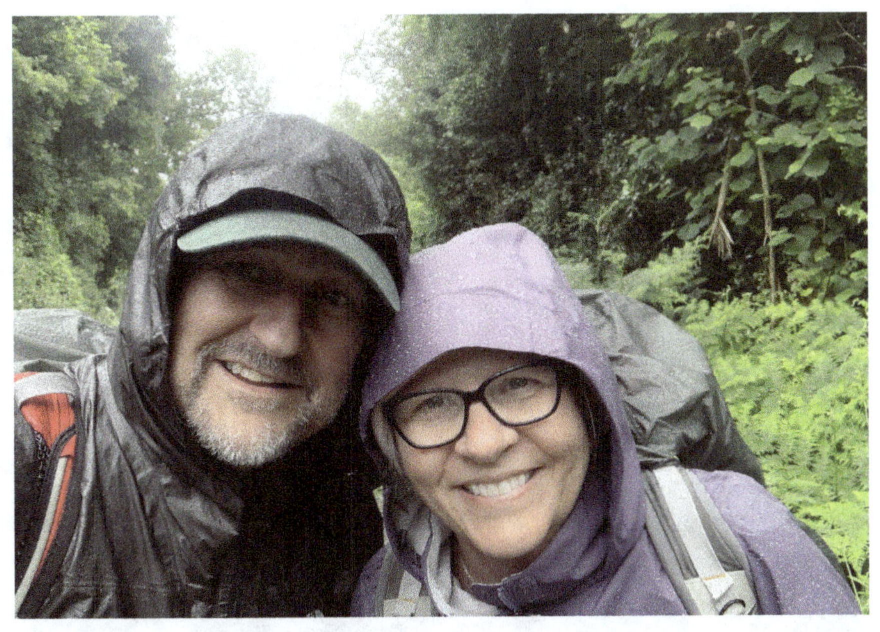

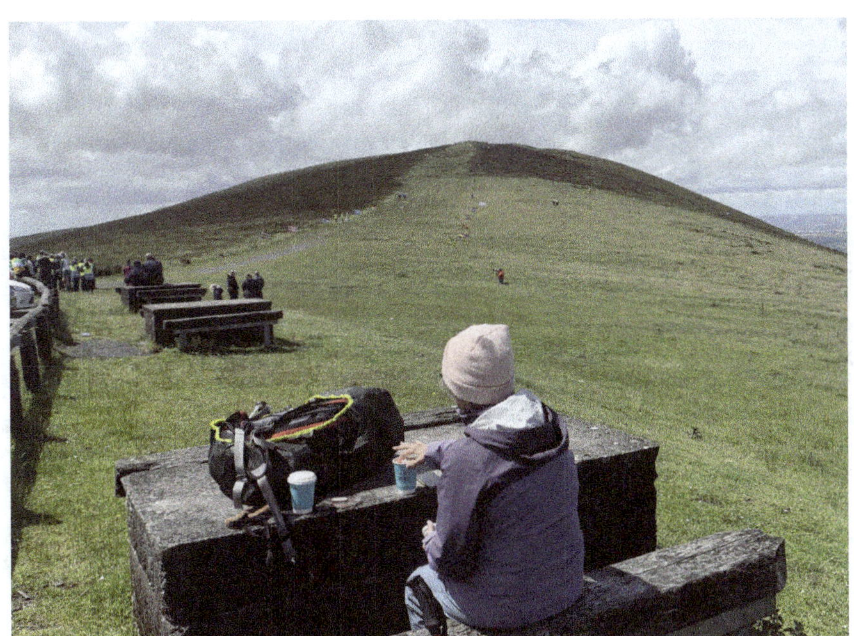

Poc Fada competition at "Nine Stones"

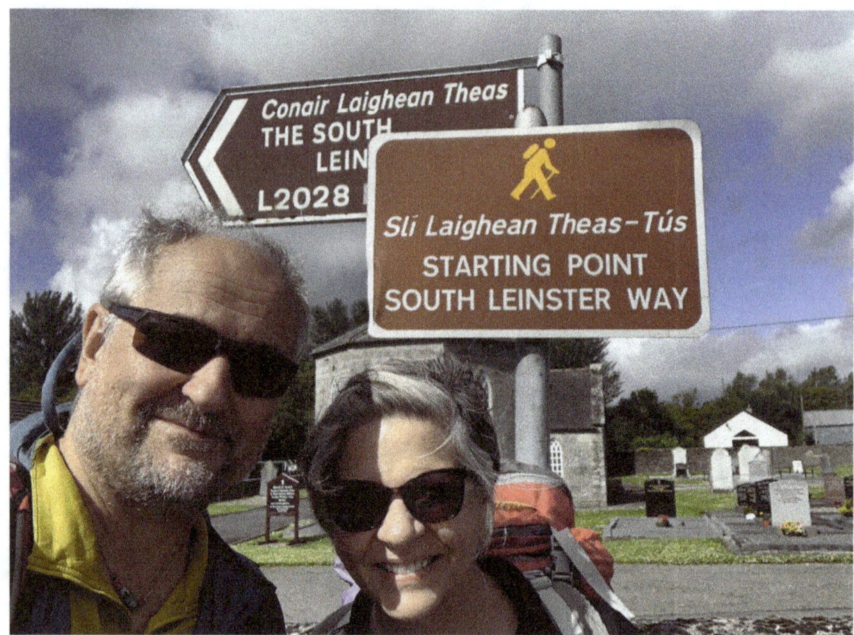

Start of South Leinster Way, Day 9

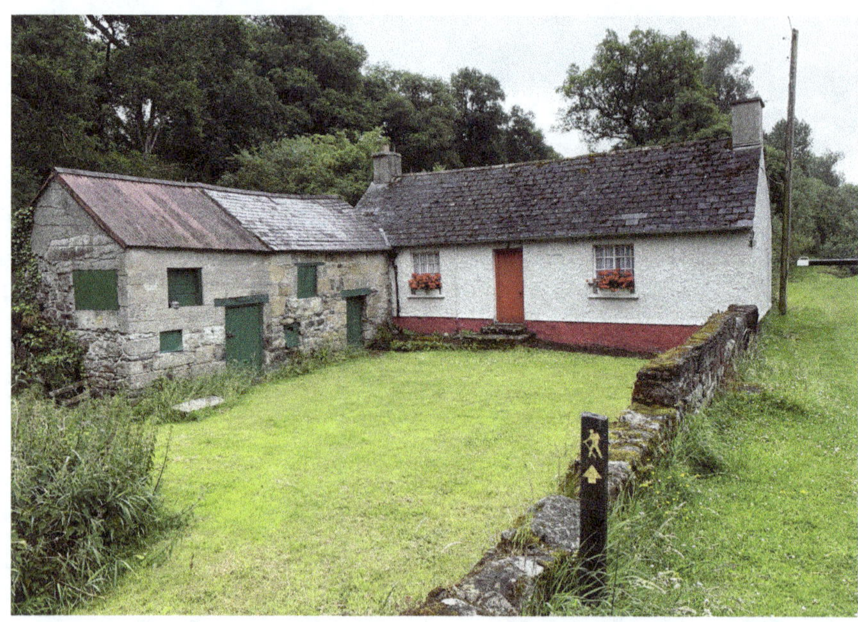

Hiking along the Barrow River, Day 10

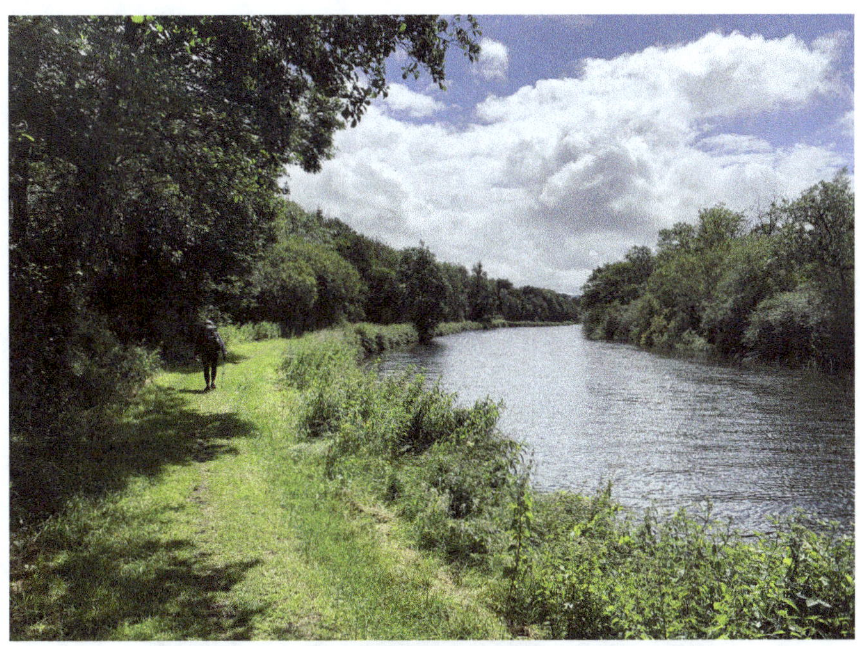

The Barrow River

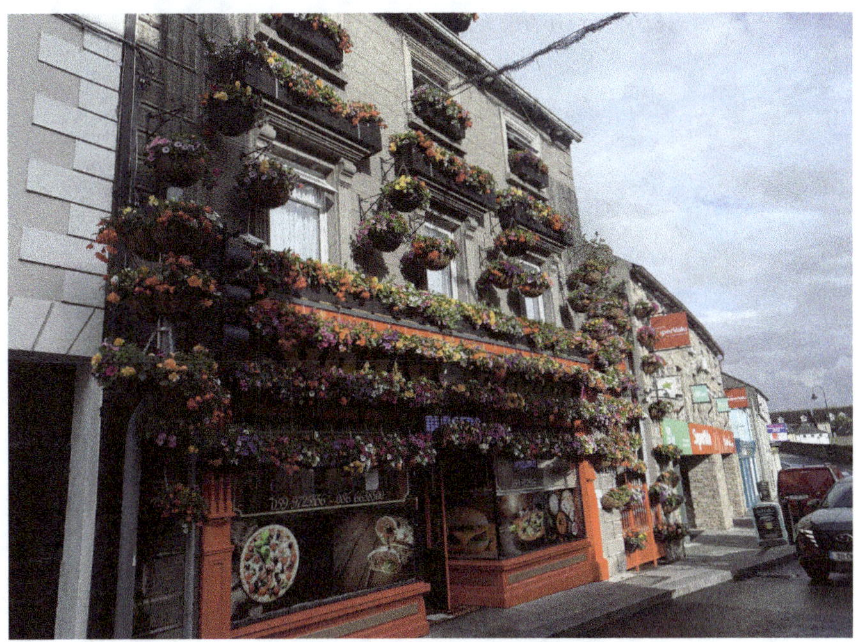

Graiguenamanagh Village

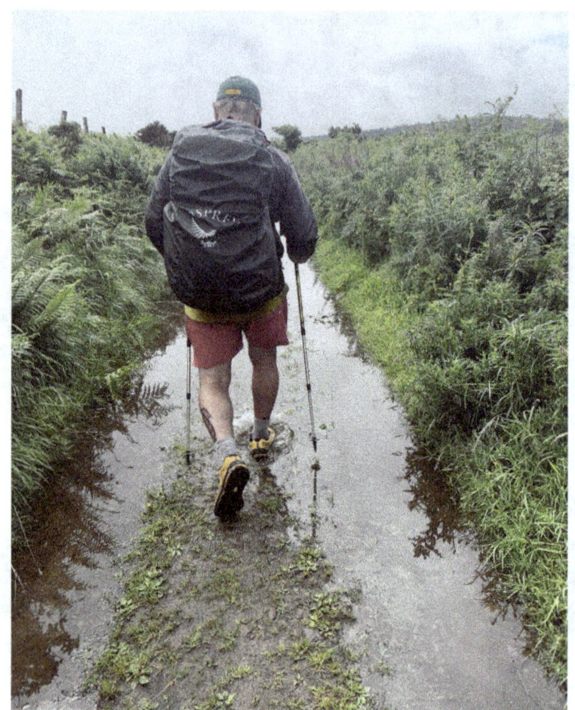

Hiking in the rain to Instioge, Day 12

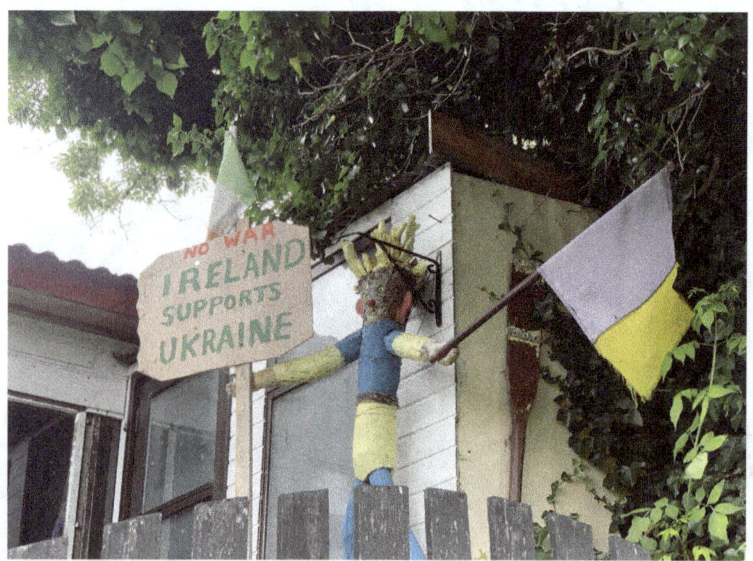

We saw lots of support for Ukraine throughout our hike

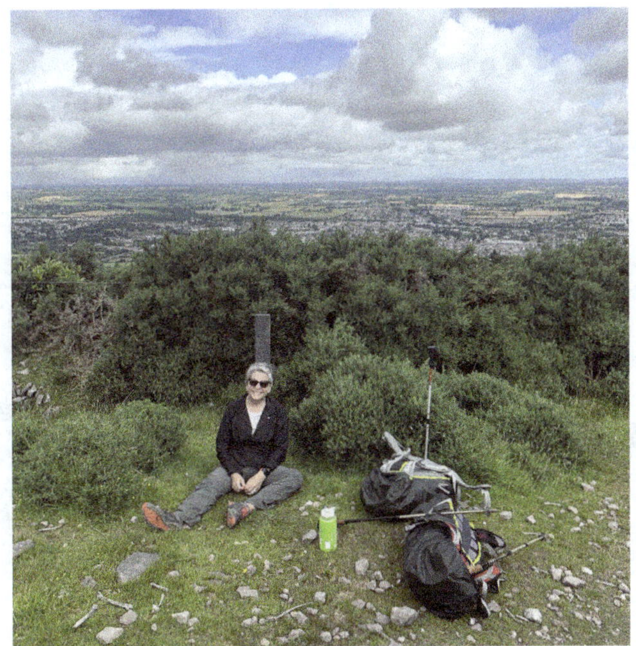

Hiking out of Clonmel, Day 16

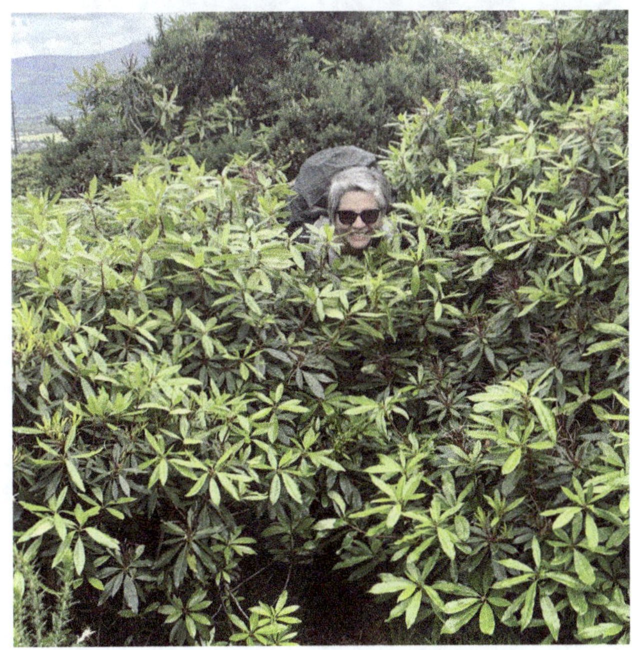

The trail has to be here somewhere

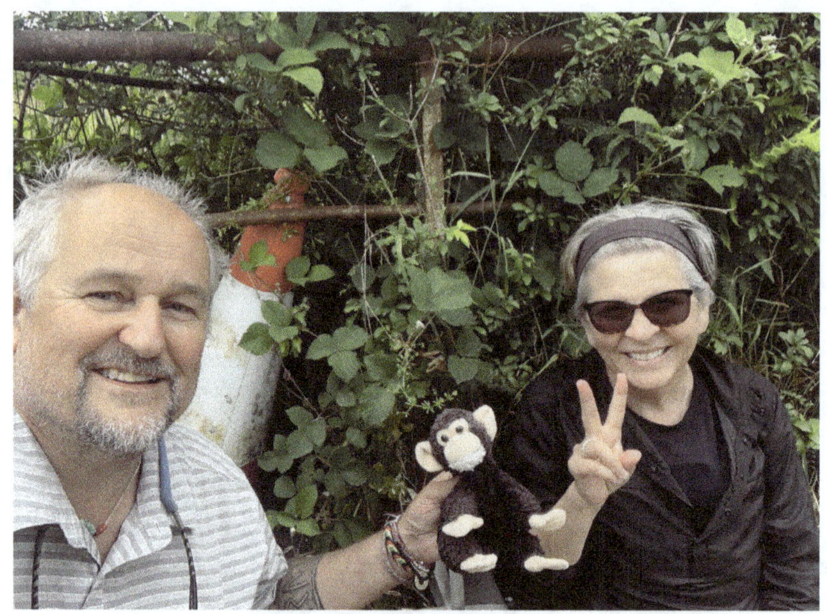

Celebrating 200 miles!

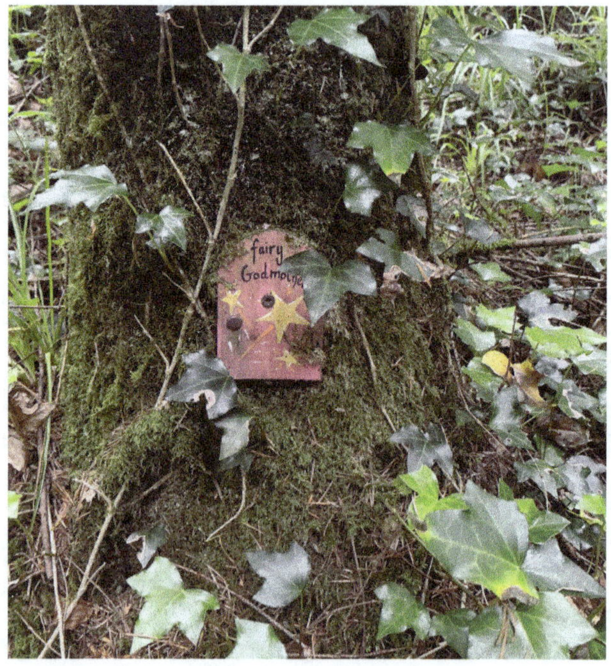

A fairy park near Kilworth, Day 19

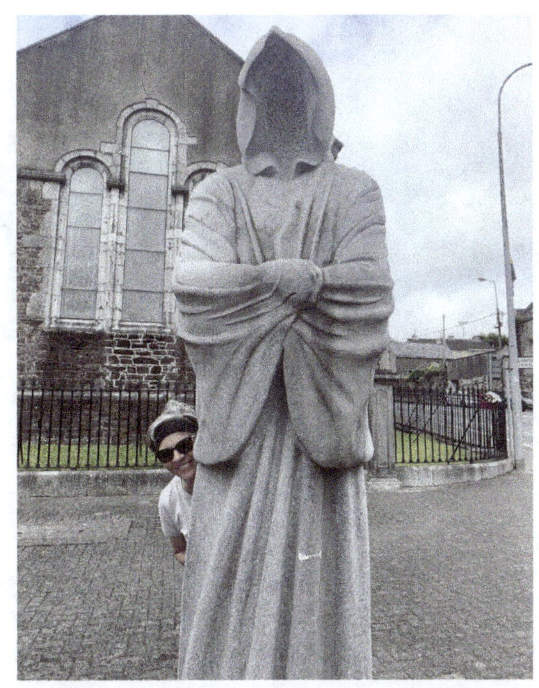

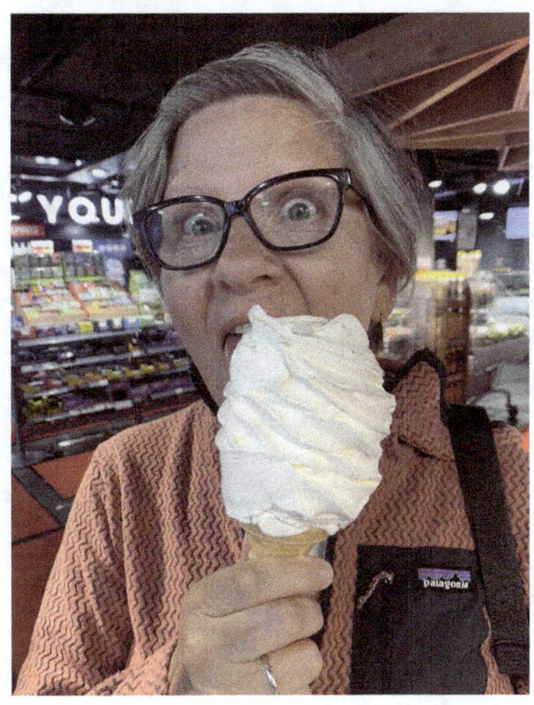

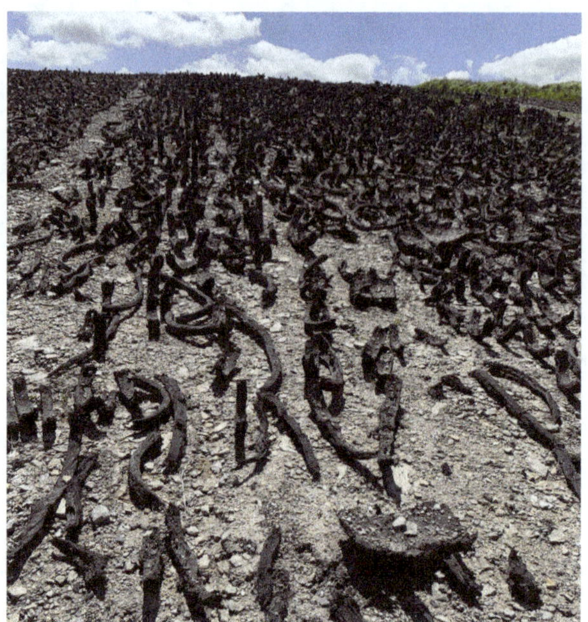

Harvesting and drying peat to burn for heat

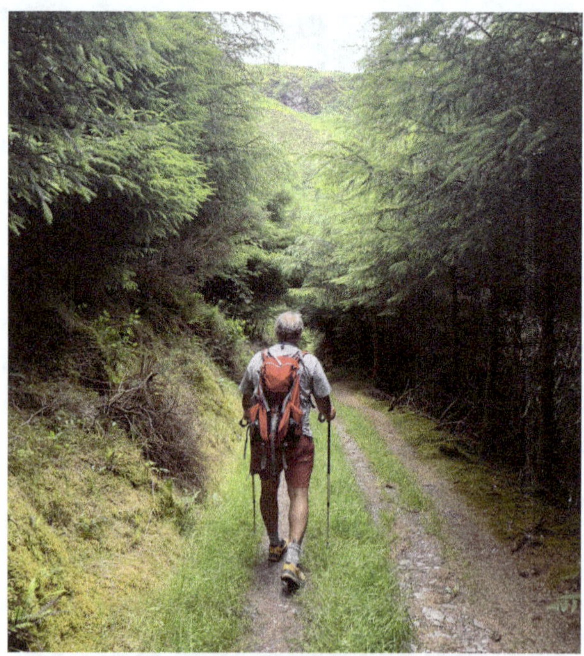

Hiking above Clonkeen, Day 25

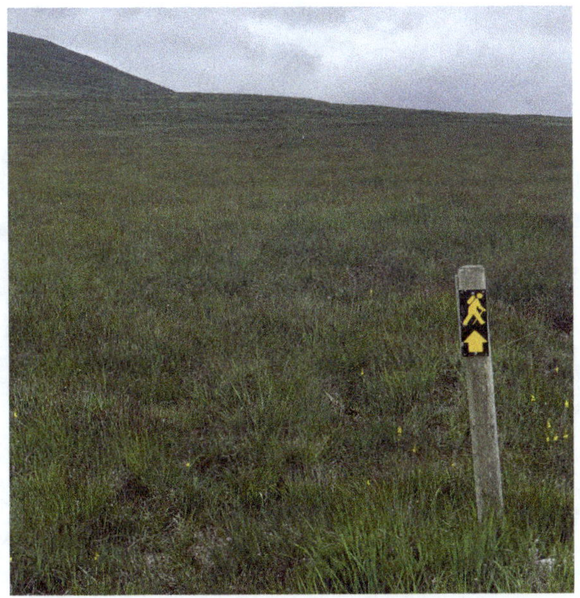

Thank God for trail signs, Day 26

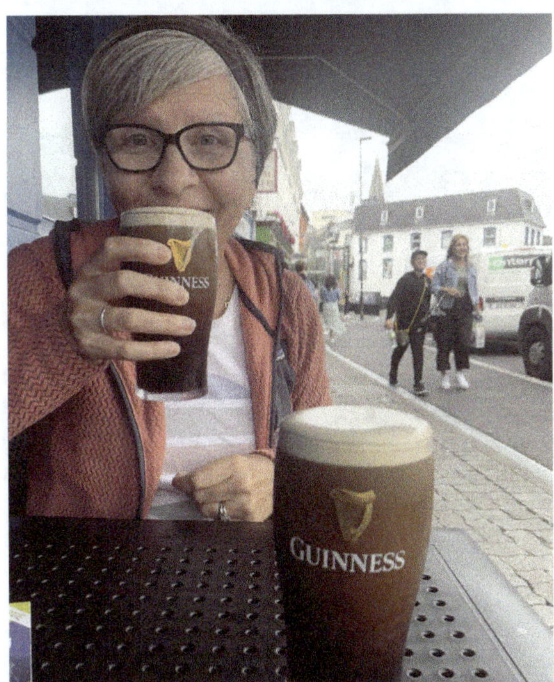

Spending the afternoon in Killarney before we start the Kerry Way

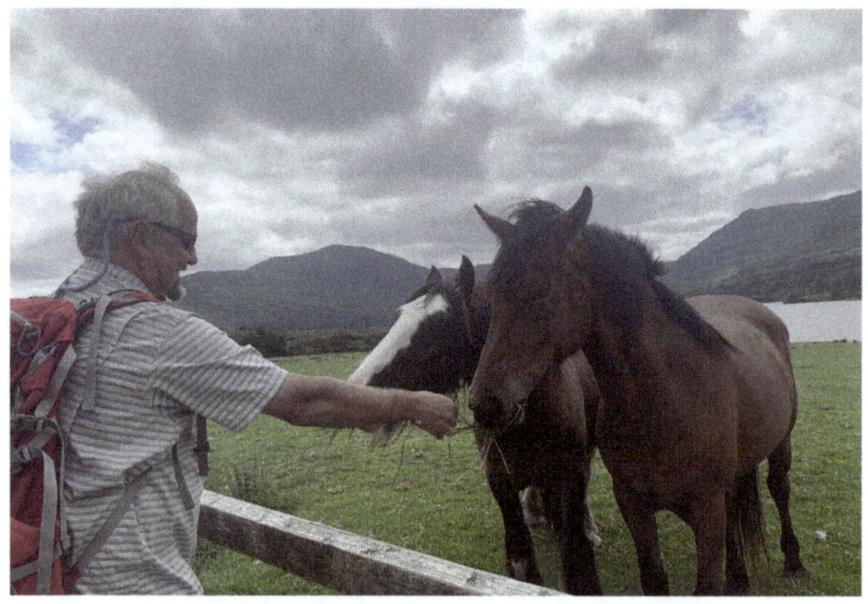

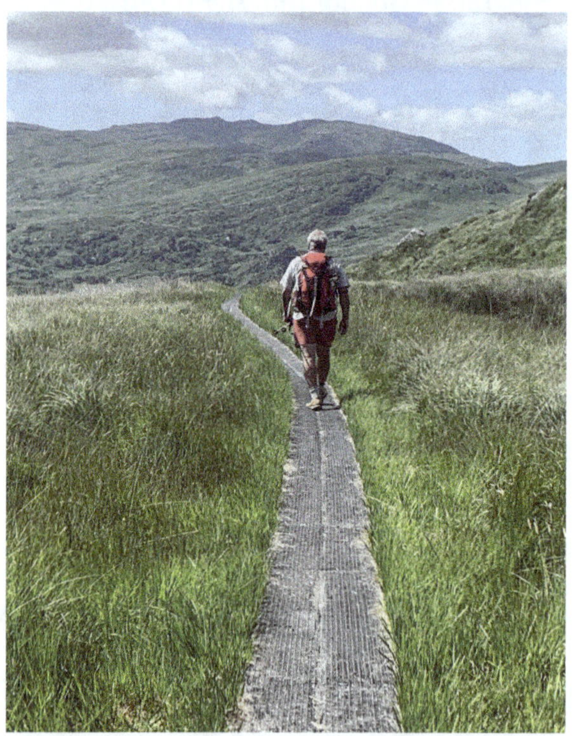

Hiking the Kerry Way, Day 28

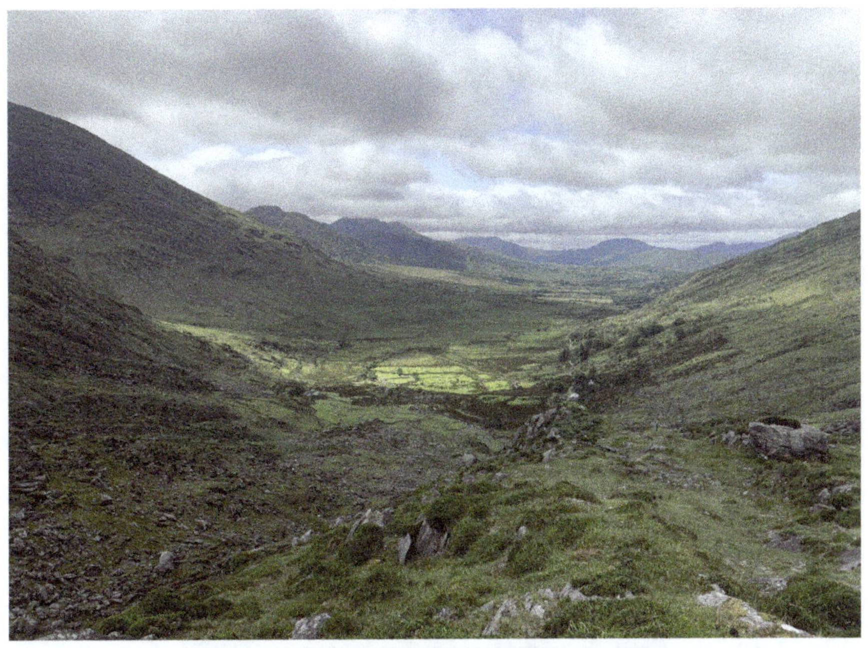

Looking into the Black Valley, Day 29

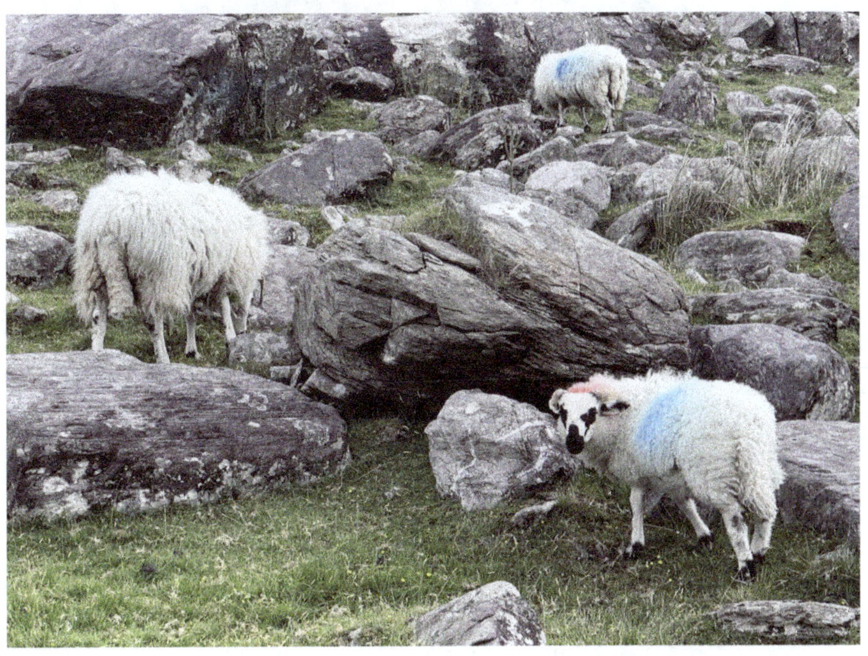

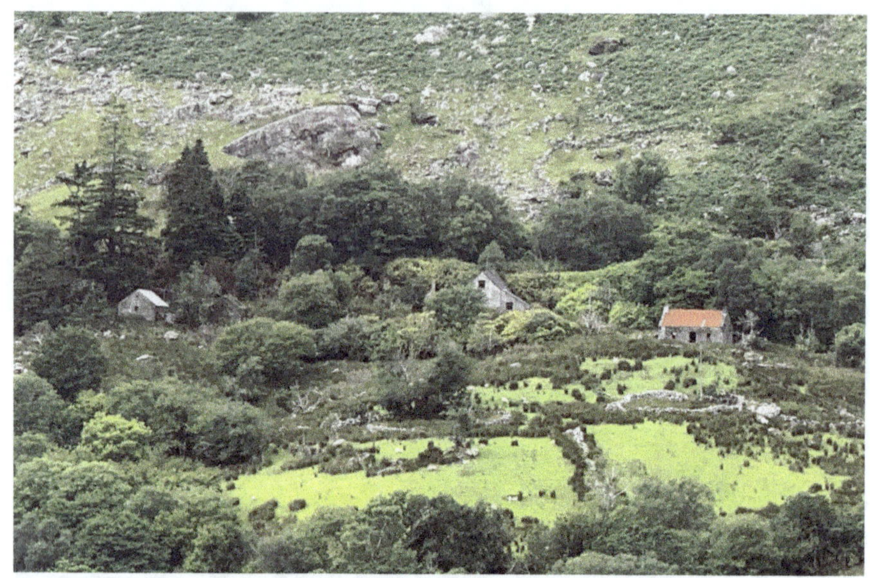

Hiking through the Black Valley on Kerry Way

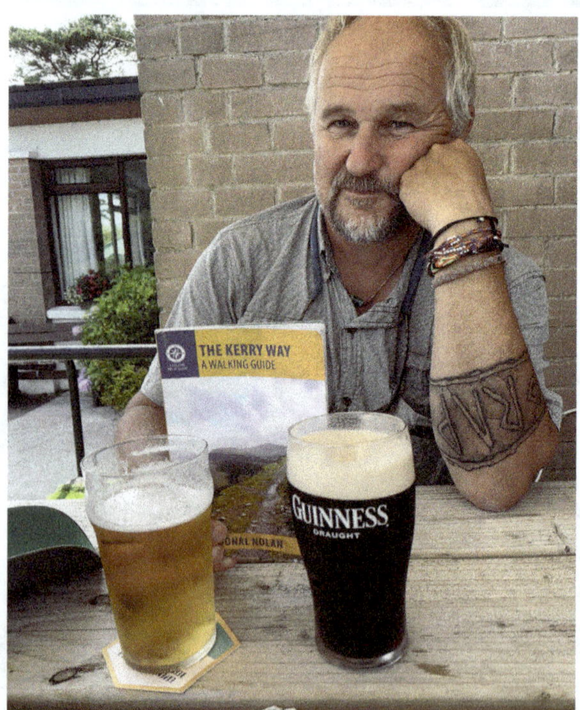

Relaxing at the Climber's Inn after a long day of hiking

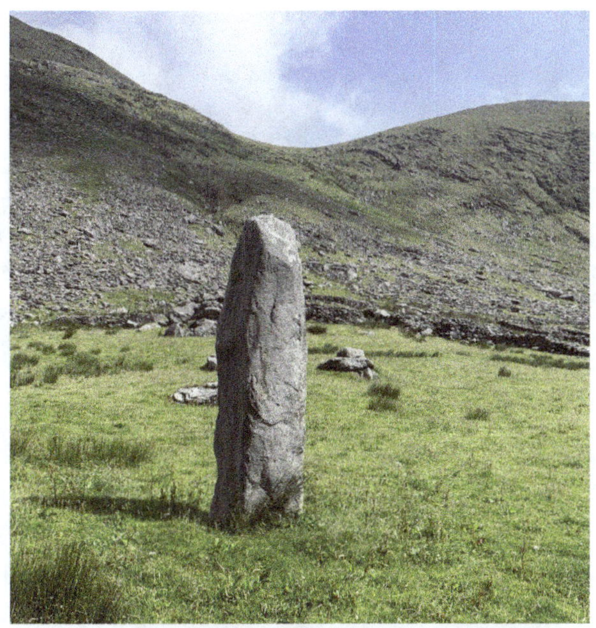

An ancient standing stone at Windy Gap

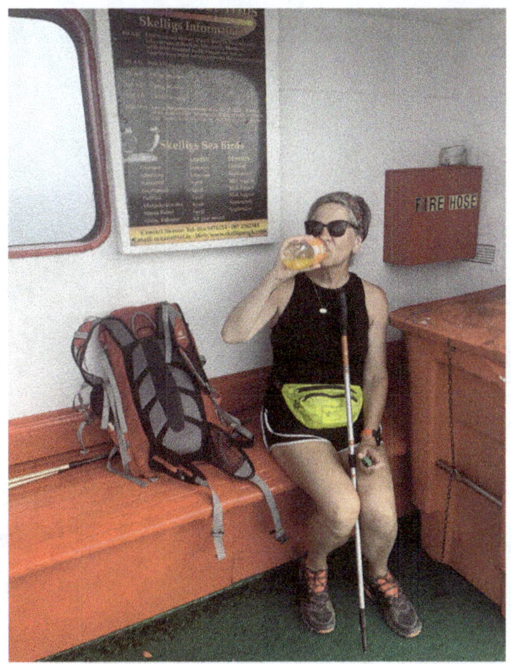

Ferry to Valentia Island on our last day of hiking, Day 32

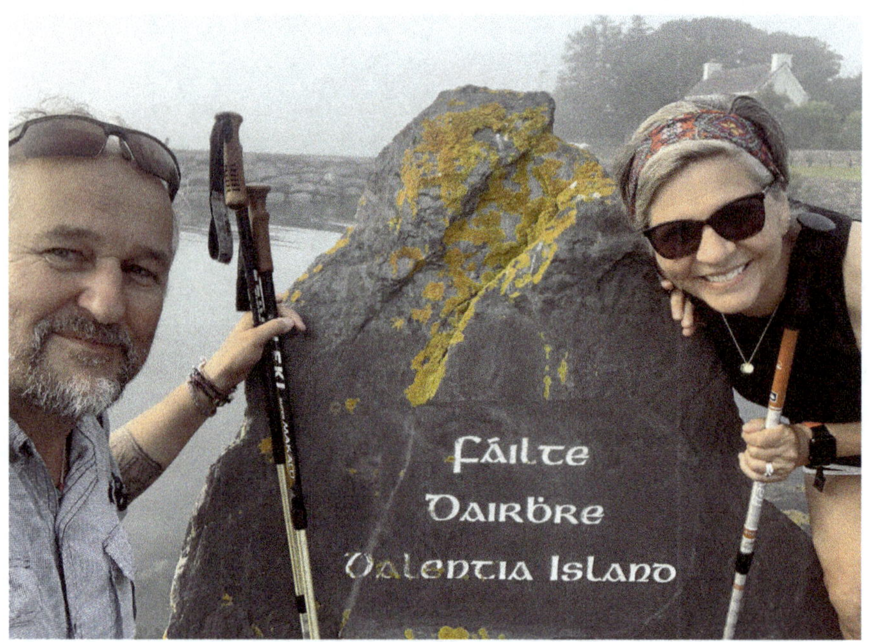

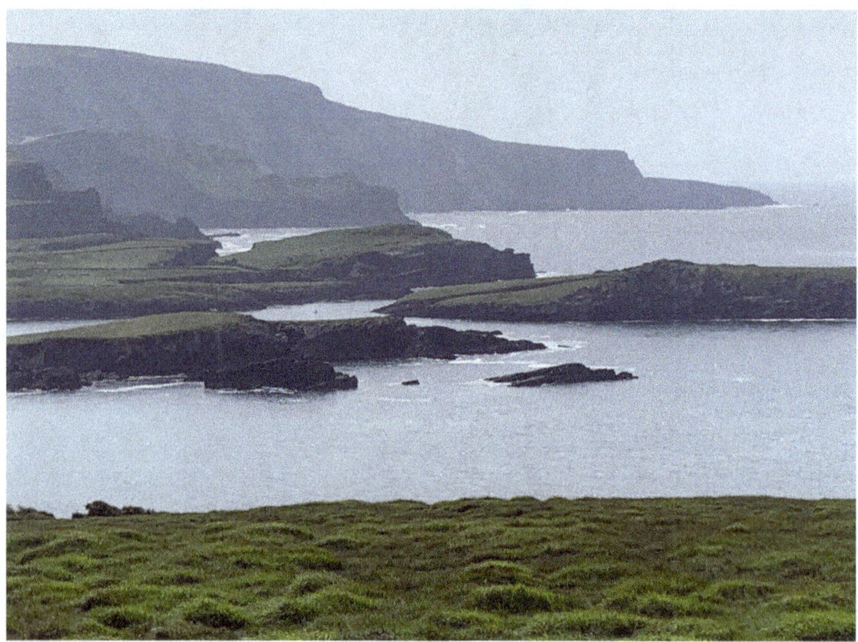

Southwest coast of Valentia Island

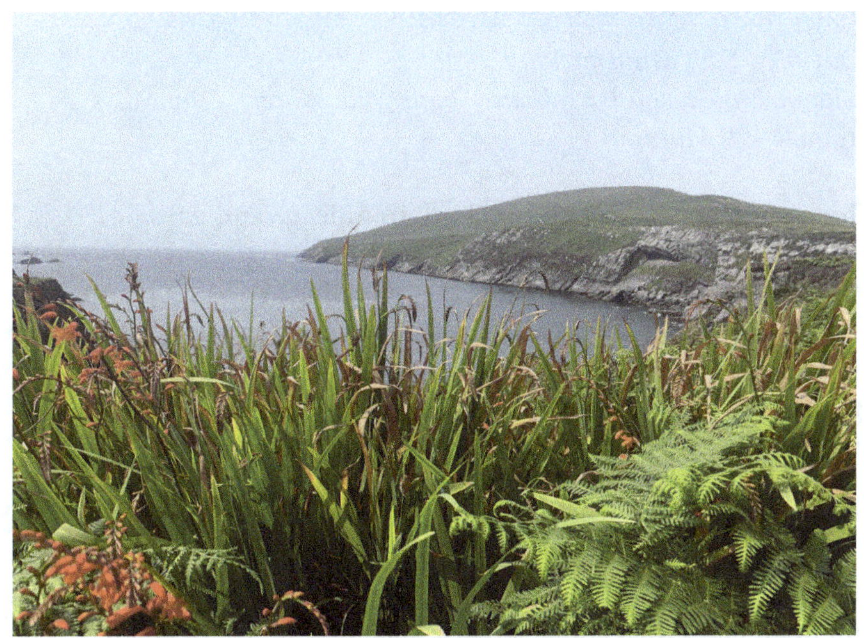

Looking towards Bray Head; The end of our 32-day hike

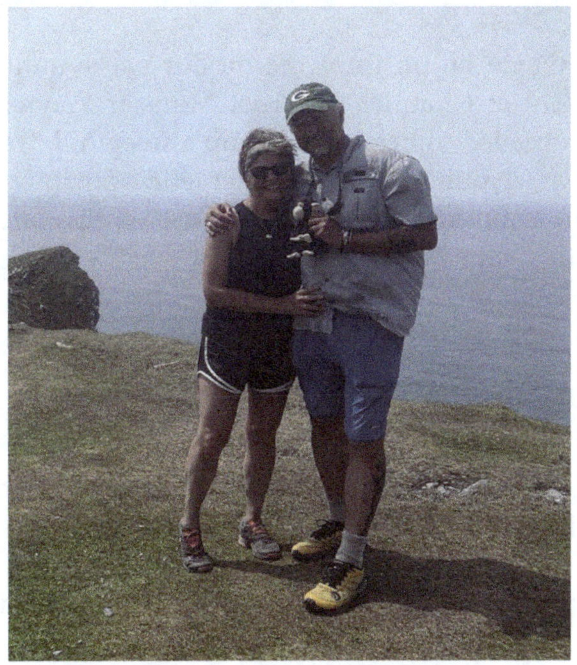

The end of a great adventure!

Day #16
Day #3 – East Munster Way
Clonmel to Glasha Farmhouse (Four Mile Water) – 9½ Miles
Total – 179 Miles

Today was our halfway point, both in mileage and days.

We had a lazy start to our day this morning. We only planned on walking 11 miles, and the owner of the farmhouse where we are staying told me on the phone the other day that she'll be at her grandson's birthday party until around 4:30pm. So, she asked us to not arrive before then.

"Walk slowly," she said.

We laid around until 9am, and then walked back over to The Hub for breakfast. Great coffee. I had a Belgian waffle with cream. Leslie had a berry scone and yogurt, her favorite meal of all time.

We somehow held off on throwing on our packs until 10:30am, and walked out of Clonmel. The East Munster Way crossed the river, and proceeded to head straight up a steep hill. As we headed out of town, a younger and very energetic woman walking and an older man standing in front of his house on this fine Saturday morning both stopped us to talk.

"Are you heading up the mountain?"

"A great day for walking."

"You should join us," I said to the old man, after he'd given us directions on which way to go.

"I already went for my long walk up the mountain this morning," he replied. This man had to be in his 80s!

Well, the narrow gravel road that headed up the mountain literally climbed straight uphill for about a mile. It was definitely our steepest climb yet. The kind of steep road where I'd be terrified to be driving uphill in a manual car wth a stick shift. Really steep.

At the top, the road turned into a gravel track and passed through a gate to the right. Within a few hundred yards, the track turned into a completely overgrown trail, a reminder that not many people hike the East Munster Way.

A worn wooden post with a painted yellow walking man, the same type of sign post that we've been following for weeks, pointed towards what looked like a sheep path that was completely grown over with tall and prickly gorse bushes and other overgrown shrubs that resembled rhododendrons. The shrubs were thick and towered over our heads.

We followed this densely overgrown and unmarked "trail" for about a quarter of a mile, not sure we were heading the right way. I lost the path a few times and had to bushwhack through the thorny bushes to find some semblance of the path again. The bushes were six to seven feet tall, just high enough to not be able to see over or through them. The hillside eventually opened up to a sheep pasture and followed along the edge of a forest. When we finally came out the other side of the thorny gorse bushes, there was no trail in sight. So, we'd lost it somewhere in the shrubs.

The paper map that I'd printed off the Internet showed a forest track that would eventually lead steeply downhill for three-quarters of a mile to a paved road. Now clearly off the marked trail, we headed in what I thought was the right general direction until we hit a barbed-wire fence and a large locked gate with several private property signs posted all over it. Definitely not the right direction.

We retraced our steps a few hundred yards, and Leslie headed off on a trail into the woods one way while I checked out a possible trail option that crossed an open area in another direction. We didn't see any little yellow walking man trail signs anywhere.

There was a dirt track that seemed to lead back down the mountain in the direction of Clonmel, so I wasn't really worried about being lost. But we'd already spent an hour just wandering around, and on Leslie's exceptionally painful feet.

Leslie found a trail that eventually turned into a wider forest track that was also heading the way that I thought we needed to go, so we made our decision.

Well . . . that track ended up winding around a hilltop, and then turned back in the wrong direction, so we cut off onto another track that led to the top of a hill, and to a big radio tower, thinking that we might be able to see the right way to go from up there and hoping that there was some kind of road heading down from the tower.

Nope.

We took a trail that seemed to be a mountain bike track, judging from the tire marks, and followed that in the general right direction for 30 minutes or so. The track had lots of big rocks and tree roots, so really did a number on Leslie's aching feet and ankles. It was slow going. I was starting to feel guilty for having lost the trail and forcing Leslie into more pain than was necessary.

The trail led downhill and hit another forest track. Just as I made my guess on which way to turn on the track, a mountain biker came zipping up from behind us. I waved him down and showed him my map. He directed us on what he thought would be the quickest way down off the mountain and back onto a road.

The best I can piece together, after the fact, is that the trail marked on the map did lead to that fenced and locked gate. So the mapped route was blocked. There were signs of charred shrubs and burnt grass all over the hillside, evidence that a fire had come through the area not long ago and had burned all of the fence posts and wooden trail signs that probably would have shown a route either around, or up and over, the locked fence.

My suggestion for other hikers on the East Munster Way would be to stay high on the hill to the left (east) of this area. Where the trail hits the dense gorse bushes, rather than pushing through them, head left and straight up to the top of the mountain to a concrete cross that is easy to see at the very top, and then down the other side bearing south-southwest.

We eventually made our way down a country road and hooked back up with the trail. But after hiking and climbing through the hills for three hours, we'd only gone a total of four and a half miles, and Leslie's feet were killing her.

We then road-walked up and down some steep but incredibly beautiful hills, and through a couple of brief rain showers, to the crossroads at Four Mile Water, a cluster of old stone houses.

Our hostess Olive, the owner of Glasha Farmhouse where we were staying for the night, was at her three-year-old grandson's birthday party. She saw us walking down the road from her son's backyard, so she jumped in her car and met us at her farmhouse just as we arrived.

Glasha Farmhouse is the nicest B&B we've ever stayed in, and Olive was probably the nicest hostess we've ever met. She has a beautiful home with several rooms for guests, with a large glassed-in sunroom where meals are served and beautifully manicured gardens. It's the kind of place that we feel funny about staying in, with our rancid clothes and backpacks. After we cleaned up, Olive served us tea and desserts in the sunroom.

She provides an amazing dinner for a fee. Since there are no other places to eat, or grocery stores anywhere nearby, we opted for the dinner that Olive was offering: three homemade breads; black and white "pudding" wrapped in Filo dough; and then an amazing salmon fillet that was super moist; potatoes and asparagus; a bottle of Rioja red wine; and a yummy baked chocolate dessert. An amazing dinner!

We enjoyed talking with the other couple who were staying there, Ray and Mary Jean from Montana. They are here flyfishing for five days. Really nice and interesting people. They travel to interesting flyfishing spots around the world.

There is a small local pub only a five-minute walk from the farmhouse, but we didn't finish dinner until 9:30pm, so we're heading straight to bed.

It was a frustrating hiking day, and a lot of work for only nine and a half miles, but we got where we needed to go. And we just had an incredible dinner tonight at the Glasha Farmhouse.

Leslie's feet are in constant, throbbing pain and she is limping with every single step. Our pace is really, really slow, but it's either that or we quit the hike. She has an amazing pain tolerance, and strong will.

Day #17
Day #4 – East Munster Way
Glasha Farmhouse (Four Mile Water) to Clogheen (Parson Green Caravan Park) – 12½ Miles
Total – 191½ Miles

Today was a day to forget.

Instead of hiking the last section of the East Munster Way, that would've been about 16 miles, we opted to road walk all day, so we'd only have to go 12 and a half. I've studied the paper maps and Google maps for several hours over the past few days, and there just isn't a way to come off the trail on this 16-mile stretch to get to any kind of road or lodging. And 16 miles in one day was out of the question with Leslie's aching feet. She's only able to walk maybe two miles per hour once her feet get "warmed up," so the distances just take longer to cover.

She's already taking the recommended limit of Advil and Tylenol every day. Her morning ankle and arch taping routine is getting a little more involved every morning, too. But it seems to be helping?

We walked on the official trail route for about two miles out of Four Mile Water, past the cute little pub, the only public building in the area.

It was cool, breezy, and overcast all day long. Rain threatened several times, but never fell. The official route of the East Muster Way continued on to a forest track, and pretty much stayed in and out of logged forest land until the final couple of miles into Clogheen.

The wide valley that we traveled west through all day was beautiful, but less scenic than if we'd been on the trail. We passed lots and lots of dairy cows, sheep, and a few horses.

We took our first break three and a half miles in at the cute little village of Newcastle. I bought a Diet 7UP and two bananas and we sat and rested a bit by the town's old water pump.

To pass the time, we played the "what color car will be passing us next" game. Correct guesses of blue, black, white, or gray scored one point each. More obscure guesses like red, yellow, green, or purple scored three points if guessed correctly. I almost always win this game. Today it lasted a while because there were very few cars on the road this Sunday morning.

Leslie jumped out to a seven to three lead, partly because she correctly guessed a red oncoming car. I clawed my way back to a seven to seven tie. And just as I was expounding on my strategy of slowly and steadily creeping back into the game, one point at a time, and not wasting my guesses on three-point colors, Leslie guessed red again and won the game 10 to seven.

She said that it was one of the happiest moments of her life.

That was pretty much the highlight of the day. We took a short lunch break of trail mix and energy bars after around six miles. And then another break at nine miles. It was slow going today, and my feet ached for a good part of the day as well.

Eleven and a half miles got us into the center of Clogheen, a cute little village with a couple of pubs, two very small grocery stores, and . . . no available lodging to spend the night, which is why we had to walk another mile out of town to Parson's Green Caravan Park, complete with a petting zoo, snack bar, horse and hay wagon rides, and a children's playground. There were lots of people camping, and then about a dozen double-wide mobile homes, one of which we'd reserved for the night.

We've passed very few campgrounds on our long-distance hikes in England, Wales, and now Ireland. But we have stayed in a couple of these caravan parks. They seem fancier and more developed than what you'd expect of a campground in the States.

We got some laundry done for just the second time in the last 17 days, and had a burger and chips at the caravan park's "chippery."

I spent a couple of hours tonight looking at upcoming mileages and options to continue walking across Ireland while trying to keep our daily mileage under 12 miles—and also trying to find lodging. The next few days we'll be passing through rural countryside, and the little villages that are near the trail don't have any places to spend the night. But, I think I have the next four nights figured out.

Tomorrow we start on the Blackwater Way, our fourth trail. We have about 14 days to go.

This evening, I put a big pot of water in the freezer for a couple of hours and then Leslie soaked her feet in the icy water, hoping it would reduce the throbbing.

Tomorrow we'll hit the 200-mile mark of our trip.

Day #18
Day #4 – East Munster Way
Day #1 – Blackwater Way
Clogheen to Montain Barrack (Lodging in Mitchelstown) –10 Miles
Total – 201½ Miles

Well, our first day on the Blackwater Way only involved walking on the actual route for about a kilometer. I decided that we need to try to limit our mileage to 10 to 12 miles a day from here on, if at all possible. Leslie's feet are in constant pain when she's not taking two Tylenol and two Advil at a time.

The trail out of Clogheen just didn't offer any options to find a place to sleep after 10 or 12 miles. My original plan was to take the trail about 12 miles, and then cut off to the south to a spot marked on the map called Aragin. But after lots of research and emailing a couple of possible lodgings, I couldn't find any place to stay anywhere near Aragin.

Instead, we opted to road-walk from the caravan park through

Clogheen for five miles to Ballyporeen, and then a little over five more miles back up to meet the Blackwater trail at Mountain Barracks crossroads. It was road walking on asphalt all day with more cars, all driving fast, and absolutely no shoulder to talk on. But 10 miles and access to a taxi at the end was better than over 14 miles to the middle of nowhere with no lodging options. It's our movie.

So, off we went.

Highlights of the Day:

- We loved our mobile home stay. We sat in the living room this morning and drank our morning coffee. I watched a little news on TV. Neither of us wanted to leave and start walking.

- About half a mile before we got to Ballyporeen at mile five, we passed a house and a guy wheeling his garbage can out to the street. He said "hello" and asked where we were heading. Neil ended up inviting us in for tea (which we didn't do) and then told us about Ballyporeen being where Ronald Reagan's grandparents lived. Neil insisted on inviting me into his house (while Leslie stood out in the driveway), while he fetched a magazine that was produced in honor of Ron and Nancy Reagan's visit back in 1980. Neil also gave me his cellphone number and told me to call if we needed a ride when we got to Mountain Barracks, or if we needed anything else. The friendliness of strangers!!

- We hit our trip's 200-mile mark today. We completely blew past our 100-mile point. We took a short break at a grassy spot just off the road we were walking along, and took a photo with Monkey Face. While sitting on our packs and celebrating with some warm water and an energy bar, we looked up and two beautiful horses had wandered over and were standing just a few feet away. Completely unnoticed. Just standing there, watching our celebration. I took a horse video for Arlo and Rio!

- We passed several large herds of dairy cows. Gerdy, the taxi driver who picked us up at Mountain Barrack crossroad to take us to Clongibbon House in Mitchelstown for the night, told us that Mitchelstown used to be known all over the world as "The Cheese Place" because of their famous local cheese. I bought some at the grocery store that we'll have for lunch tomorrow.

Low Points of the Day:

- Leslie started moaning about midnight last night because her feet ached so bad. She took two Advil so she could at least get some sleep.

- Our pace is really slow these past few days. Maybe miles an hour at the most. So, it just takes much longer to get anywhere. I know Leslie is gutting it out and in a lot of pain. I'm carrying her water bottle and all of our snacks and lunch food just to lessen her pack weight a little bit.

- We barely said ten words to each other during our hike today. I just think Leslie is concentrating on keeping her legs moving. I know she was close to tears several times today.

- We stopped for our snack break in Ballyporeen at a picnic table in front of the Ronald Reagan Center. It's a very small museum honoring his ancestors and his visit. When we sat down for a break, Leslie said, "Everyone is excited to tell us about their Reagan connection and we didn't even like the guy."

Two More Highlights:

- When we got to Mitchelstown and the Clongibbon House, we dropped our packs in the lobby and went across the street to Dexy's Bar, a little pub that served locally brewed microbrews from Eight Degrees Brewing. The Eight Degrees IPA that was on tap was amazing!! And, the bartender, Dexy, came over and sat with us for a while. He told us about a partnership between Jameson Distillery and Eight Degrees Brewery to produce some whiskeys aged in IPA kegs and in stout kegs. I'll see if I can find a bottle in Dublin before we head home.

- Chili Tandoori: the best Indian food either of us have ever had!! Mind blowing!! Definitely worth coming off the Blackwater Way to Mitchelstown for. It really was the best we've ever had.

Eight in the evening. . . . Relaxing in bed. One day at a time. It's all we can do.

Day #19
Day #2 – Blackwater Way
Mountain Barracks to Fermoy – 10 Miles
Total – 211½ Miles

After our hike today, we're back at Dexy's Bar for more locally brewed beer. This time there were seven or eight local guys, all but one drinking Guinness. Leslie mentioned that a couple of the guys ordered two pints at a time.

Robert was sitting off to the side by himself, and he seemed very drunk. It was only 6pm. His head sort of bobbed up and down, like he was falling asleep. At one point, he staggered his way to the bathroom, but couldn't negotiate the bathroom door to get inside.

After a while, Robert looked our way and asked, clear as a bell, "What part of the States are you from?" and then proceeded to tell us three of the funniest stories about his time in the States. He said he'd lived there on and off for the past 25 years.

The guys at the bar were laughing right along with us, and egging Robert on. "Tell them about the time you got arrested." "Tell them the one about getting kicked out of the same bar twice in one night."

Needing no encouragement, Robert told us how he got a job as a semitruck driver in Nashville, Tennessee. He ended every story with a smile and a twinkle in his eye, and said, "You gotta laugh. You have to enjoy life. It's important to laugh." The guys in the bar listened and laughed, even though they'd probably heard Robert's stories hundreds of times. A bit of a celebrity, having been a local guy who lived and worked in the U.S. for much of his adult life.

As we drained our beers and got up to head to dinner, Robert stood and shook our hands and offered to buys us a drink. Just as I was ready to say, "Sure, I'll take a shot of Jameson," Leslie piped up and said we were heading to dinner, but thanks for the offer. Grrrrrrr.

We had a much better hiking day today. We left our packs at the Clongibbon House so Leslie hiked packless, and I just had a dapack with food, water, and a few other things. We hiked only 10 miles on mostly level ground and gentle hills. And the first six miles were on a nice forested track. Leslie's feet still ached, but not as badly. Trail walking with no pack puts less pressure on her feet.

We haven't really figured out what is up with Leslie's aching feet. She has hiked around 1,500 miles on our last two long-distance hikes with no problems other than blisters and occasional shin splints. It's likely the hiking shoes she chose for this hike that started the issues, and we just haven't rested the several days necessary to help her feet heal.

The forest hiking was quiet. And as we started off from the Mountain Barrack crossroads, where Gerdy the taxi driver dropped us back off this morning, the surrounding hills were covered in a misty cloud that formed water droplets on our arms and clothes as we walked along. It felt good to be back in the forest.

There were tons of flowers all over in the open areas and in the clear cuts. The mist and trees and flowers felt magical.

The trail came out of the woods at a car park just outside of Kilworth. We noticed one, then two, and then dozens of little four-inch by four-inch wooden signs, each nailed to the base of the trees lining the path. The first sign we bent down to read said something about entering a "fairy park." Some were painted doorways for fairies to enter at the base of a tree; some had names painted on them. An entire section of forest full of little fairy signs. One said, "Fairies gather here after dark."

The Blackwater Way then followed some very busy roadways into the large town of Fermoy. We were going to end our hike today at the Forge Bar and Restaurant, but it was closed when we got there, so we called Gerdy to pick us up and bring us back to Mitchelstown.

Dinner at the Hunter's Rest.

During our taxi ride home, Gerdy talked a bit of politics. He's not a fan of Sinn Féin. He said that the young Irish are all getting caught up in their promises of equity, and helping poor people. Gerdy said that the current leader of Sinn Féin was quoted as saying that she admired Fidel Castro. "I think they are all Marxist," Gerdy said. "They're being led down a dangerous path."

I disagreed, but only in my head. It seems like a lot of the older Irish we've met fear any changes that look like "socialism," and have a deep-rooted fear of immigrants. Gerdy didn't mention immigrants specifically, but he had that flavor to his comments.

Earlier today, we walked by large "castle" remnants that we later learned were just fortified houses of rich landowners from back in the 1500 and 1600s. Back then, it was one large family or clan fighting another for land. And then everyone was fighting the invading British. Gerdy showed us where huge British military garrisons and barracks used to be before they were destroyed by Sinn Féin after Ireland won its independence. "A shame that all of those buildings were destroyed. A tragedy," Gerdy commented.

Day #20
Day #3 – Blackwater Way
Fermoy to Killavullen Loop Trailhead – 14½ Miles
Total – 226 Miles

Just a long damn day!

We hiked without our packs today.

We paid 125€ (!!!) to transport our packs from Mitchelstown to Mallow.

Shocker, I know.

We'd arranged for the bag transfer with Gerdy knowing that we were going hike about 15 miles today. He wasn't available to do the transfer, but he arranged for another taxi driver to pick us up at our hotel in Mitchelstown this morning at 9am. I should've known when she pulled up in a fancy 15-passenger minibus that it was going to be expensive.

The driver brought us down to Fermoy to start where we'd left off yesterday, and then was going to transport our backpacks to the Hibernia Hotel in Mallow later today.

"How much all together?" I asked.

"You need to pay me now."

"Or course. Of course. How much will it be all together?"

"125 euros."

Gulp.

Our hike started by heading out of Fermoy along the sidewalk and then the roadside for a mile or so. Early on we were passed by two older (one very overweight) morning walkers.

Leslie's limp seemed more noticeable to me this morning than the last few days. I asked her about it, and she said she was just getting warmed up.

Just outside of town, we headed up a forest track and into the woods. All day today the route rotated between forest track, dirt trail, and narrow, untraveled, and hilly rural roads.

About halfway through the hike we realized that even on the rural roads we hadn't seen a car the whole time. Just five or six big tractors.

The trail passed through rolling hills, but not nearly as high or steep as the previous week.

Cool and breezy.

Overcast.

It seemed like it was on the verge of raining all day, but the clouds never opened up. We live by the weather. I regularly check a couple of different weather apps, paying close attention to the clouds, wind direction, and speed.

Despite the long walking day, it was a really pleasant hike on the Blackwater Way. We crossed several small creeks, and passed horses, cows, and farm after farm after farm.

Our goal for our lunch break was the eight-mile point at a road crossing into Ballyhooly. We walked another half-mile past that crossing and picked a grassy spot along a narrow road, across from a horseback riding trailhead. There was an empty car attached to an empty horse trailer that was parked across the road from where we stopped. Someone out riding for the day.

My butt cheeks had been chaffing badly for the past few miles, probably from a combination of sweat and poor hygiene. As soon as we stopped, I grabbed our small plastic container of Vaseline and dropped my shorts to my knees to apply some much needed lubricant.

Just as I was pulling my pants back up, the car across the street pulled away. Apparently someone had been inside the whole time, and got a pretty decent show of my white butt.

It's my mom's 90th birthday today! We called and sang "Happy Birthday" in the classic Wunrow, two-part harmony. Leslie and I practiced our parts a couple of times while we walked today, but when it came time for the actual performance on the phone our harmony fell apart and we had to start over.

We passed a couple more fortress towers that were likely part of an old family estate, and some really beautiful views of the surrounding area. We also continued to pass a surprising number of old and newer abandoned homes and farms. Like, dozens over the course of the day. Some are partial constructions that were never completed, and others just seem to be abandoned. COVID? Housing crash? Economy slump? Every time we hiked past an unfinished house, I'd think about what I would do to fix it up.

Our hike ended at a trailhead for the Killavullen Loop Trail, and then we walked about three-quarters of a mile into the village of Killavullen to the only establishment in town . . . wait for it . . . an Irish pub. Of course. It was called the Haven Bar.

Four locals and the bartender all greeted us as we walked in. Leslie got a cider and I got a pint of Guinness. The guys were all friendly and asked about our trip. The backpacks we carried inside gave us away.

I asked the bartender if he could help us call a taxi out of Mallow to come get us. "That will be tough. Taxis won't come out here. I guess they don't like our money," he replied. He called a couple of taxis, but they declined. And then one of the guys got out his cellphone and called a different company, who said they'd be out to get us in 20 minutes.

I offered to buy a round for everyone, as a thank you for their help. One of the guys said, "In this bar, if you buy me one, then I need to buy you one. And I don't think you want to stay here all night." The bartender asked if I wanted a "half-Guinness" since I'd finished my pint.

"Sure," I replied.

As I handed him some money, he said, "No need to pay. We appreciate what you and your wife are doing."

We got dinner at a grocery store after settling in at our lodging in Mallow. Some slices of chicken and ham, fresh bread, olives, humus, and Mitchelstown's "Famous Cheese" that I've been carrying around since Mitchelstown. It was a nice change from restaurant food.

We were both exhausted and fell right to sleep. Leslie said her stomach felt funny when she went to bed. Might have been the "Famous Cheese."

Zero Day
Mallow – Hibernian Hotel

Well . . .

Leslie got up at least five times during the night to throw up. Something in her stomach needed to get out of there. She said she felt fine otherwise, but just couldn't keep anything down. She tried a sip of water at 3am, and that came right back up.

So, we took a well-deserved day off.

By the end of the day, Leslie was sipping Diet 7UP and was able to keep a banana and scone down.

I went to the post office and mailed home some maps and Leslie's down jacket, got more Advil and Paracetamol at a pharmacy, and got our laundry done. I had dinner all by myself at a place down the street. It felt lonely.

I eat out by myself when I travel, all the time, but after spending every minute of the last 23 days together, I found myself missing Leslie after just being apart for an hour.

Day #21
Day #4 – Blackwater Way
Killavullen Loop Trailhead to Ballynamona – 10 Miles
Total – 236 Miles

Leslie woke up feeling much better. She wasn't really hungry, but had some coffee, yogurt, and fruit for breakfast.

Taking a day off from hiking seemed to really help her feet. Still some pain and a slight limp, but Leslie said that the day off worked wonders.

We hiked at close to a normal pace all day (without packs), and Leslie only took one dose of Advil and Paracetamol today.

After hiking 10 miles through the hills, we both felt great. Like we could have gone on forever. Granted, it was with no pack for Leslie, and a light daypack for me, but we could both tell that hiking the last 20 days has gotten our legs and bodies in much better shape.

We got back to the hotel by 3pm, and it felt like we hadn't even done anything today. This hiking without packs is nice.

The 10 miles from Killavullen to Ballynamona was a great hike. An equal mix of rural roads, forest track, and overgrown foot trails. It surprised me how overgrown with tall grass and bracken the actual Blackwater Trail was. Very unused. We missed a turn in the trail, twice, because the small signpost was partially covered with tall vegetation. We haven't seen a single hiker on this trail over the past few days.

At one point, we were on a wide forest track (like a rural tractor road) and the track made a sharp right turn, heading straight up a steep climb. Within 100 yards, I was like, "This doesn't seem right," so I backtracked and found a covered up trail signpost and the overgrown trail that we'd walked right past. Few to no hikers and no trail maintenance on the Blackwater Way.

The weather today, and what is forecast for the next week, is amazing: low 70s and sunny with just a few clouds. Light breeze. Classic Ireland weather . . . just kidding. Even the locals have been marveling at the nice stretch of weather that we're in the middle of.

It's our third night at the Hibernian Hotel. It's starting to feel like we live here. It'll be nice to move on tomorrow. When I emailed the Donasheka House B&B to make a reservation a few days ago, I told the host that we planned to walk to the village of Nadd and wondered if there was any transportation to her place from Nadd (hoping she'd take the hint and offer to come pick us up).

No luck.

She replied that we should really have our own vehicle if we want to stay at the Donasheka. I've adjusted our hiking route to take us way off the Blackwater Way for the next two days so we can get to places to stay in a reasonable amount of walking.

After we take the trail to Bweeng tomorrow, we'll head off-trail for a day and a half. Choosing the best route across this part of Ireland is all about being able to find lodging at the end of the day, or ending in a place where we are close enough to a big enough town that it will have a taxi to help get us from the trail to lodging and back again in the morning. These next two days on the official Blackwater Way have neither towns nor taxis. So, we'll improvise.

It's 7pm and the skies are clear and sunny. Our room is hot from the sun. We're laying around in our underwear trying to stay cool.

With only nine days or so left of our cross-Ireland hike, I started making some lodging bookings since I know that the upcoming Kerry Way will be busy, and lodging near the trail will be booked.

My mind has been drifting to home, and responsibilities. I said again to Leslie as we were hiking today, "Enjoy the scenery. Enjoy the peace and quiet. Enjoy this simplified lifestyle. Because soon enough, we'll be back home and wishing we were still out here."

Day #22
Day #5 – Blackwater Way (Day #1 – Duhallow Way)
Ballynamona to Laharn Crossroads (Donasheka House B&B) –
11½ Miles
Total – 247½ Miles

Heat wave!!

We heard on the news this morning:

"A heat wave is covering Ireland."

"Extreme temperatures cause a health warning."

"Parents are encouraged to keep their children indoors."

And the high today was only supposed to hit 76 degrees!!

Keep your red-haired, fair-skinned Irish children indoors!!

The first six and a half miles from Ballynamona to Bweeng was on the well-signed Blackwater Way, but it was all road walking. Once again, more tractors than cars on the road. Even though it's a Saturday, farmers are cutting hay and silage, and contractors are bailing up the silage in huge black plastic wrapped bales. The hay will lay out in the sun for several more days to dry out before its bailed.

It felt really hot by 11:30am when we started walking. We started late on purpose because our B&B for tonight doesn't allow check-in until after 6pm. I think it's because they are a working farm. We'd gotten our hopes up that the "Chippie Snack Wagon" we saw in an Internet photo parked in front of the Bweeng Pub would be open when we got there around 2pm. We'd envisioned an icy Diet Coke and something to eat. But the Chippie Snack Wagon didn't open until 5pm. So disappointing!

Instead we sat in the shade of a stone wall a couple blocks away and ate our ever-evolving bag of trail mix that we keep adding ingredients to, plus two bananas and some left over Doritos from the other day.

I tried to complain about the 75-degree heat that felt like 85 degrees to me, but Leslie wouldn't have it. A couple of times I said I'd much rather be walking in cold wind and rain than in this heat and relentless sun. Leslie shut me down. "Just enjoy the day and appreciate the scenery," Leslie reminded me several times, to my total annoyance.

Our packs seemed heavier to both of us today. Probably because we are coming off of a day off, followed by a day of hiking without our big packs. And since our B&B tonight is in the middle of nowhere, we're also carrying lunch for today and tomorrow and dinner for tonight. Plus, we each added a bottle of an Irish version of Gatorade to our packs along with a full liter of water for each of us. Two liters of liquid adds over four pounds to each pack. And we needed the extra liquids in the heat today.

About a mile north of Bweeng, the Blackwater Way turns left and heads into the woods. We continued instead on a narrow, untraveled country road another three and a half miles to Laharn Crossroads because it is the closest lodging we could find to this section of the trail—and we are nowhere near a town big enough to have a taxi.

Leslie's feet were feeling a lot better today. The heavier packs while walking on pavement all day today may ruin them, but she made it through the entire day on two doses of Advil and Tylenol instead of three or four. Tomorrow, we have another longer road-walking day to meet back up with the Blackwater Way trail, so she might be totally lame again by then.

Early on in our hike today, a guy pulled up and rolled his window down to ask if we wanted any water or tea. It was already hot outside, and he'd probably heard the same warnings we did about keeping the kids indoors.

And then again in Bweeng, when we were sitting up against a stone wall resting and eating our lunch in the shade of the wall, a lady and her two little kids and dog named Coco stopped to see if we needed anything. She said that when she came back past us in a half hour, she'd give us a ride to our B&B. Total stranger.

So nice!

Leslie said again that she plans to be a nicer person when we get home.

We arrived at the Laharn Crossroads about 5pm and had an hour to kill before arriving for the 6pm check-in at Donasheka House.

We'd cooked up in our minds that the owners were mean, crabby, and unwelcoming. We concocted all sorts of dialogue about how they would likely shun us for our odor, and not appreciate our effort to get to their B&B (miles off the trail). Our fictional welcome was all because of the email we received saying that we probably shouldn't consider staying there since we didn't have a car, and couldn't check in until 6pm.

Laharn Crossroads has a little park-like spot with some benches, a tiny bandshell, and an outdoor wooden dance area with a posted sign that said, "Person Dancing at Own Risk."

Google describes this park location as "Laharn Criss-Cross Road Dancing." There is a sign that says dances are held every Sunday night from eight to 10, with a different band each Sunday. That's tomorrow night, so we'll miss it. But it sounds interesting and unique . . . and to be honest, something we'd likely never do.

We walked uphill about five minutes to arrive at Donasheka House right at 6pm. Nora was outside watering some potted plants. We were stunned by the view from their house and out across the valley. It seemed like you could see forever.

Nora welcomed us into her farmhouse, and asked if we wanted tea and dessert now or to freshen up first and get settled in.

After showers, we joined Nora downstairs in her living room full of her own paintings and beautiful china in two large cabinets. She brought us each a slice of apple pie and a pot of tea. "The pie isn't very sweet because we don't eat much sugar in our house," said Nora. I thought it was delicious, and I hoped for a second piece that never arrived.

Nora was the most engaging and funny person we've met on this trip! Our premeditated assessment of what she would be like couldn't have been more off base.

Nora made a point of using our names frequently as we talked, and directed questions to each of us. It would take several pages to recount the things we talked about over the next two hours!!

We started with Irish politics.

I asked Nora lots of questions about their president, Michael Higgins, who is apparently well-loved all across the country, and about the Irish "Taoiseach," Leo Varadkar, the equivalent of a Prime Minister for the country. I used the title, "Prime Minister" several times in the conversation, and each time Nora corrected me and said, "Taoiseach."

We talked about reunification with Northern Ireland, someday, and Nora was eager to hear our views on Donald Trump and Joe Biden. She wondered how the U.S. could ever have elected Trump, and why the U.S. is so in love with guns and violence? Questions that we couldn't answer, because we don't understand it either.

We shared Nora's disgust with Trump, gun proliferation, and violence in the U.S. We told Nora that these are difficult questions for us to answer as well.

We covered the British royalty. Nora is convinced that Megan Markle has brainwashed Prince Harry to leave the royal family.

We learned a lot about how Ireland currently has a coalition government that does not include Sinn Féin, but that Sinn Féin is gaining in popularity and will likely be in charge in the next few years. Nora said, "I don't care if someone is Communist or Democratic, as long as they are helping people."

Nora kept referring to the Green Party as the "Vegetable" party, and their current party leader as the "Little Vegetable Man."

Nora's husband, John Joe, joined us after about an hour. He'd been on his tractor all day cutting grass for silage. He asked lots of questions about where we're heading and where we've been. John Joe said he hates walking, and couldn't believe that we walk all day, every day, and were walking across Ireland. He kiddingly said he doesn't even like walking down his driveway to get the mail. He's a tractor guy.

Nora and John Joe have never had any guests walk to their B&B. They were particularly intrigued with the fact that we'd walked all the way from Dublin to their house.

It was rare for us to sit and talk with folks for an entire evening. But it was fun.

At 9pm, we went upstairs to our room realizing that we hadn't had any dinner. We made a couple of peanut butter and jelly sandwiches from hard rolls and jelly that I took from breakfast this morning. I also made a little salami sandwich from the salami that I've been carrying for days. I used the rest of our bread to make sandwiches for lunch tomorrow.

Day #23
Day #6 - Blackwater Way (Day #2 – Duhallow Way)
Laharn Crossroads to Mahon's Rock (Millstreet) – 13 Miles
Total – 260½ Miles

In Bweeng, we switched from being on the Avonhu Way, part of the Blackwater Way, to the Duhallow Way part. Both of these trails combine to what is referred to as the Blackwater Way. I actually read a sign yesterday that was posted in Bweeng at the start of the Duhallow section that said that the Munster Way refers to everything between the Wicklow Way and the Kerry Way. So, the South Leinster Way, Munster Way, and Blackwater Way. That's the one and only time I've seen that designation.

After about four miles of country road walking, we arrived in the village of Nadd. There's something about that town name that makes me chuckle.

We needed to get back to the Duhallow Trail (Blackwater Way) after diverting up to Laharn Cross for our lodging with Nora and John Joe last night.

There wasn't any coffee setup at our farmhouse room this morning, so I just mixed up a couple of instant coffee packets that we've been carrying with us in a drinking glass of lukewarm water. Leslie turned her nose up at my concoction, but who got the caffeine withdrawl headache this morning? Not me.

Last night, as we chatted in Nora's parlor, she asked whether we'd seen any "fairy forts" yet? We told her about the little fairy signs and tiny doorways that we've seen in the woods along the trail a few times. "Are they fairy forts," I asked. Nora said that fairy forts are a group of trees that were purposely planted in a circle hundreds of years ago as a place for fairies to live. She said that they have little tunnels and underground rooms. These old fairy forts are protected by the Irish government and cannot be cut down or molested in any way. Nora said that local people will not even enter a fairy fort for fear of triggering bad luck.

This got us into a conversation about superstitions. Nora said that many people who live in the countryside, especially older folks, are very superstitious. And these superstitions vary from county to county. Nora shared a couple: if you enter the house through the front door, you must leave through the back door; or, if two table knives are inadvertently crossed, one on top of the other, it means bad luck will come.

We knew today was going to be another hot hiking day. And it delivered. Close to 80 degrees, no clouds, and almost no breeze. We roasted!! Even though we were walking by 9:30am, it already felt warm and a little muggy. The sun seems really intense in Ireland and it was often hard to find shady spots to get out of the sun for a break.

Out of Nadd, we followed a narrow road that climbed for about three straight miles. We stopped at a bridge that led into a massive wind farm for lunch because there was a nice breeze. I'd pre-made some peanut butter and jelly sandwiches and we had an orange and some of our bottomless trail mix.

Then we followed a dirt path uphill and hit the Duhallow Way trail. It always feels good to be back on the official trail.

For a couple of miles, the trail led through old peat bogs where long, thin chunks of peat were cut out of pits by hand or by a peat cutting machine. These strips of peat are laid out to dry for several weeks, and then collected and cut up to burn in the winter as stove fuel. Peat harvesting in this bog has been going on for hundreds of years.

We met a local guy out for a long walk in the afternoon who explained that as a kid his parents had him working in these peat bogs, cutting peat blocks all summer long. He said that each local family has a right, or a permit, to cut in a specific designated section. And that families have been cutting in their designated sections for hundreds of years.

These days, there is some kind of tractor attachment that scoops up big buckets of peat when it is still moist and mushy and squirts it through this strainer attachment to create long strings of peat that are maybe three inches in diameter. These long strings of peat are then left in the sun to dry. We saw these "fields" of drying peat all over the place. The peat chunks/strings get hand-turned a few times before they are collected and taken home to burn for fuel.

Our 13-mile hiking destination today showed up on the map as "Mahon's Rock" with a little parking area in front. When we eventually got to the main road that led to Mahon's Rock and then on into the town of Millstreet, I called a taxi to meet us at Mahon's Rock in an hour and a half. I had a hard time describing to the driver exactly where we'd be waiting. The driver, John, had never heard of Mahon's Rock, or more likely I was just mispronouncing it. It took three different phone calls, then he said he'd call me back to confirm where we'd be waiting.

We didn't know at the time that the final mile led straight up a steep hill in the blistering sun, climbing a thousand feet in elevation over just a mile. And we were out of water.

When John finally arrived we both thanked him profusely for getting us out of the sun. John said, "Just happy that you're safe."

Our B&B in Millstreet, the Knockerish, is about a quarter of a mile out of town. And our room is tiny—two single beds that we can barely squeeze around. The shower is so small that when I dropped the soap, there wasn't enough room to bend down to pick it up.

Our room was super hot and stuffy when we arrived. The sun was shining in through the big windows and as we've realized several times, windows in Irish homes only open a couple of inches. It was impossible to get any air moving.

Noreen, our B&B hostess, was very friendly and funny. She offered us a ride into town for dinner since it was a bit of a walk from her place.

Leslie and I were both more tired at the end of today than we have been on any day so far on this hike. Thirteen miles is a long way to go through the hills with backpacks on, but it was the heat and relentless sun that really got us today.

Day #24
Day #7 - Blackwater Way (Day #3 – Duhallow Way)
Mahon's Rock (Millstreet) to Croohig's Cross – 11 Miles
Total – 271½ Miles

Okay, I'll admit it. I've become kind of obsessed with standing stones.

Our maps denote hundreds of little markings that say "standing stones," "row of stones," "circle of stones," and occasionally, "Neo-lithic Tomb." We passed several standing stones today . . . basically a tall stone that is sticking up out of the ground in the middle of a field. They are usually pretty narrow or slender, and definitely not naturally occurring.

Nora told us the other day that they were erected hundreds of years ago by chieftains who ruled over a section of land. And if a chieftain had more than one stone, or a row of stones, it was a sign of wealth or power. We saw several stone rows and a couple of circles of stones on our walk around Wales. I'm enamored with them, and am constantly on the lookout.

I think I'm intrigued simply because they are so old. Knowing that people erected these "signposts" centuries ago. I just looked them up on Google, and here's what I found:

> *Standing stones, called "Menhirs," are tall, upright stones erected in pre-historic times. The single stones, as opposed to stone rows or circles, marked grave sites, land borders, routes, and perpetuated important people's memories. Stones in lines were likely calendar constellations to mark important points in the Celtic course of the year. Circle stones were most likely used to practice rituals and ceremonies.*

Stone circles date back to between 4600 BC and 6000 BC!!

Many of the stone burial chambers in Ireland are older than the pyramids!!

Anyway, I'm going to keep watching for them along our hike.

It was supposed to be as hot today as it was yesterday, so we loaded up our two liter water bottles, and each carried two sports drinks. But at the top of the mountain pass at Mahon's Rock, where we were dropped off this morning at 9:30am, it was windy, cold, and blanketed in heavy fog. I loved it!

We quickly walked out of the fog, but a decent breeze kept up all day long. The sky stayed cloudy, too, so it never felt too hot.

The last five miles of our hike to Croohig's Crossing climbed and then wound around Claragh Mountain, first through a dense pine forest, along a pine needle covered path, and then through tall grasses along a barely discernable trail. We both remarked that the Duhallow Way is also not well traveled, just like our last few "Ways."

We saw one guy out for a walk on the trail today, but that was it. Once again, we haven't seen any through-hikers or section-hikers since we were on the Wicklow Way weeks ago.

The trail continued through a sheep meadow. It reminded me of walking around the coast of Wales. No real track, but the trail was very well signed, so no chance of taking a wrong turn. It was a really pleasant second half of the hike today.

Earlier in the day, as we walked through downtown Millstreet, we stopped for a water and snack break at a covered bench in front of a big church. An aged, stooped Catholic priest, complete with a pressed black shirt, white clerical collar, and black sweat pants, walked up to say hello. He had to be in his 80s, at least. He saw my backpack and said, "Are you heading up to the mountain? When I was a boy, we used to run to the top of that mountain every day."

Dang.

He told us that he had been a parish priest in Nebraska for 47 years and was a big Cornhusker fan. Having spent most of his life in the States, he was happy to come home and spend his final years in Ireland.

At the end of our hike, when we got to Croohig's Crossing, which was just a crossroads about four miles southwest of Millstreet, we called our taxi guy, John. He couldn't come to get us for an hour, so he gave us the number of another taxi guy, also named John.

When John #2 showed up, he said that people called him "Bob" to keep him straight from the other John. His dad's name was Bob, and everyone in town knew his dad. He said that it was just easier to go by Bob.

I told Bob about John Joe. He guessed that John Joe's actual name is probably Joe, but his dad's or grandpa's name was John, so he's known as John Joe, or "John's Joe."

Tomorrow is going to be a hard day. Thirteen miles with lots of uphill. There's also some rain in the forecast for the morning.

We had a little picnic for dinner at a small park next to our B&B. Chicken wraps, Doritos, and fruit. It was a nice change from restaurant and pub food.

Day #25
Day #8 - Blackwater Way (Day #4 – Duhallow Way)
Croohig's Cross to Clonkeen (End of Duhallow Way) – 12 Miles Total – 283½ Miles

Really beautiful hike today.

By far my favorite day of the whole hike.

Today we hiked the final section of the Duhallow/Blackwater Way. The final 12 miles. The high point was hiking a couple of miles through the Shrone Moore, a high, treeless boggy area surrounding the peaks we were traversing. The tall grass was wet from last night's rain.

We dropped off a gravel road and into a grassy meadow, and then across a creek. Without posted trail signs, there was absolutely no evidence of a trail. No path at all, just lots of tall grass. We headed what seemed like the right direction, and walked uphill for quite a while. The heat from the last few days have brought out billions of flies, and they surrounded us as we hiked . . . driving me crazy. Every few seconds, I smacked my arms, legs, or neck and would always kill four or five flies with every swat. That's how thick they were.

The trail then headed into heather, and the views opened up. We could see the "Paps" (two large mountains) up ahead. The heather was super uneven, and tough to move through, hiding thousands of ankle-twisting holes. It was slow but beautiful hiking through the high heather meadows.

Again, there was no evidence of an actual trail, but we could see trail signposts spread out across the hillside ahead. It was super slow walking due to the holes and hillocks and occasional hidden rocks, but the scenery was breathtaking.

We eventually dropped down to a narrow gravel road that led through a stunning valley below the eastern Pap, whose summit was covered by clouds. I read on an interpretive sign that at the top of both of the Paps is a prehistoric cairn that is 12 feet by 50 feet in size and were burial sites or "passage graves." Even from a mile or more away, we could see these stone cairns atop the mountains.

We sat on a patch of grass next to the beautiful Shrone Lake and had some lunch.

These last few miles of the Duhallow Way provided an unexpectedly beautiful piece of trail.

We climbed up out of the valley and then walked on a narrow paved roadway for the final four or five miles of the Duhallow that led to a cluster of houses and a church in an area known as Clonkeen, and the end of this section of the trail.

It remained cool and overcast all day long, with a nice constant breeze whenever we were out of the trees.

The Blackwater Way ends rather unceremoniously at a bus stop on highway N22 where we called a Killarney taxi to come pick us up. We drove the road into Killarney that we will be walking tomorrow. It's 11 to 12 miles from the end of the Blackwater Way to the start of the Kerry Way. The two trails don't connect, so we'll road walk tomorrow to hook the two together for our through-hike.

We arrived in the very busy city of Killarney. Our taxi driver, Shane, said that although there are more tourists in Killarney now than in the past two COVID years, there are still significantly fewer than in the years prior. It seemed super busy and touristy to me.

We took showers and then sat outside in front of Dan Linehan's Pub and people-watched while we drank a Guinness. Then I walked to Lana's, an Asian fusion restaurant and got takeout.

And now we're watching the latest installment of the hearings from January 6th.

Day #26
Road Walking to Connect the Blackwater Way with the Kerry Way
Clonkeen to Killarney – 11½ Miles
Total – 295 Miles

Since there isn't a designated trail that connects the end of the Blackwater/Dunhallow Way in Clonkeen to the start of the Kerry

Way in Killarney, today's 11-plus miles were all road walking to get from one the end of our fourth trail to the start of our fifth.

Leslie initially was like, "Why don't we just take a taxi, since we're just committed to hiking these five trails?" I am on the side of, "We're hiking across Ireland, not hiking and getting rides across Ireland." She gets it, but still brought it up a few more times. I think she's just testing my resolve, and don't think she would actually take a ride.

Our taxi from Clonkeen into Killarney with Shane yesterday afternoon brought the topic up again as he asked us what we were doing and where we were going. And Shane got it right off the bat. He said, "Of course you are going back tomorrow morning to walk the Clonkeen to Killarney section. You're not going to cheat. Even if no one else knows, you'll always know."

Thank you, Shane.

We wanted to get these 11 and a half miles of road walking out of the way, so it could feel like we had the afternoon off. We got our taxi at 8:30am and were walking out of Clonkeen at N22 by 9am.

N22 was super busy with really fast moving cars and semis. We were mentally prepared, but it still wasn't fun. Huge semis whipping past with a constant parade of cars and not much of a road-side to walk on.

We had to walk about five and a half miles on N22 before we could cut off onto a country backroad in Glenflesk that ended up going past a large lake, Lough Guitane. The lake was at the base of some beautiful surrounding mountains. A nice surprise. We had our lunch—some old trail snacks—while sitting in a grassy cow pasture overlooking the lake.

It was a relatively "quick" 11 and a half miles to Abbey Cross, the crossroads where we connect to the Kerry Way, about two miles south of Killarney.

After calling a taxi for a ride back to the Failte Hotel for our second night, we dropped our packs and poles and wandered around downtown in touristy Killarney, first grabbing some lunch and then doing some souvenir shopping. We only ended up getting some gifts for our grandchildren—a little hurling stick and sliotar for Arlo, and cute Ireland T-shirts for Arlo and Rio.

Leslie bought some Irish chocolate. I packed it all up with some maps we no longer needed and a couple of books we'd read along the way that I didn't want to get rid of. I stuffed everything into a very large padded mailer and mailed it all home.

Our evening was the usual: sitting in bed reading emails and Internet news on our laptop and iPad, reading our books, and journaling until we couldn't keep our eyes open any longer . . . 8:30pm. I enjoyed a bedtime snack of canned pears and some milk.

Day #27
Day #1 Kerry Way
Killarney (Abbey Cross) to Hillcrest Farmhouse (Black Valley) – 11½ Miles
Total – 306½ Miles

We passed the 300-mile mark today without evening knowing it. When Leslie and I hiked our first long-distance trail together, the Southwest Coast path in 2015, we had a little celebration at each 100-mile mark. All the way past 800 miles. I guess that novelty has worn off.

It was an amazing hiking day today, and we are both beat. The Kerry Way lived up to its billing as one of the most spectacular hiking trails in Ireland. We're staying at the Hillcrest Farmhouse that is perched on a rocky hillside in the stunning Black Valley, known as the most isolated, uninhabited place in Ireland. I'm anxious to talk with the owner about what it's like to live here year-round.

We walked up to the front door of the farmhouse around 3:30pm, and were greeted by a fairly old lady wearing an N95 mask.

She said, "Hello. Did you have a good walk?"

"Yes, it was great."

"You are in Room #4 up the stairs. Dinner will be at 6pm."

Leslie pointed to a small room with a table to the left of the stairs, "Is that were dinner will be?"

"Yes."

We carried our packs up the steep, narrow farmhouse stairs to Room #4, and Leslie said, "That's what I like. A no-nonsense welcome."

Passing through the last several miles, I was glad that we'd requested dinner when we made our reservation for tonight since there are no villages or stores for miles in any direction.

The Kerry Way starts on a busy paved path. Busy with people out for a stroll, a few joggers, bikers, and several horse-drawn "jaunting cars" (buggies) filled with tourists. The trail first passes along scenic and huge Lough Leane and through Killarney National Park.

The first few miles were flat and flew by, with lots to see and to anticipate: lake views, Muckross House (a massive mansion built in 1443); Muckross Abbey (a ruined monastery built in 1848 by a Gaelic chieftain); and then on past Torc Waterfall, Ireland's best known waterfall according to our guidebook, *The Kerry Way: A Walking Guide* by Donal Nolan.

At the base of the waterfall, the trail climbs up a steep path through an oak forest and then spills out into the wide open rocky slopes of the Torc Mountains.

It seemed like just a few seconds before we'd been on a busy paved path, and now suddenly we were out in the middle of nowhere following a foot trail through heather-clad slopes and incredible scenery.

We saw a couple dozen day hikers along the way. Maybe 10 or so looked like their packs were big enough to be hiking the entire 11 miles to Black Valley.

Just above the Torc Falls, we met Karen from New Jersey standing next to her massive backpack at a trail crossroad, confused about which way to go. We figured it out together, and then walked and talked for about 45 minutes. Karen was hiking the entire Kerry Way and carrying her tent, sleeping bag, pad, etc. I watched as she hoisted her pack onto her back, and I was glad our packs were only 25 to 30 pounds.

After walking and talking for a bit as we ambled along the trail, Leslie and I opted for our first break of the day and told Karen that we'd likely see her again along the trail.

Parts of the trail today were really rocky, which did a number on our ankles and knees. Overall, it was a great hike. Around 11 miles in, we got to Lord Brandon's Cottage. I'd seen it on the map months ago when I was planning this trip, but didn't realize until I read this section of our guidebook while walking today that it had a café! So, that motivated us onward, as we conjured up visions of cold Guinness or a cider. Unfortunately, the menu only had pop and juice. But we still took advantage of the picnic tables to take a well-deserved rest. We sat in the shade and drank ice cold Coke Zeros and had a nice long break.

A couple times toward the end of our hike today, we passed a family—mom, dad, and two teenage kids—who had hired a guide to lead them on a day hike of this first part of the Kerry Way. This seemed a little weird to me since the trail is so well traveled and signed. But the mom and dad were both pretty overweight. The mom looked severely sunburned, and was just limping along. The guide, a guy about our age, was all fit and trim and would hike ahead with the kids and then stand and wait, with his hands on his hips, for the overweight parents to catch up. They all seemed a little depressed to me.

It's 5:30pm. A half-hour until dinner. This B&B offers a fish dinner for 26 euros each. Pricey, but we are literally in the middle of nowhere. The only other things within miles of us are the Blackwater Hostel, a church, and another B&B. Instead of carrying a dinner with us, consisting of some bullshit from the SPAR grocery, we'll have a nice dinner served to us tonight.

Can't wait.

While I'm writing, Leslie is dog shopping on some Humane Society web page in Indiana. She's obsessed with getting a new dog since or beloved Goldie died a few months ago.

Salmon, potatoes, carrots mashed up with some kind of white veggie, broccoli, apple pie with fresh-made cream on top, and tea! Really good homemade cooking. Nothing fancy.

I asked Mary if she could make us something for lunch tomorrow and she said she could do a ham and cheese sandwich with an orange. We're set. There is literally nothing in the way of food between here and where we'll end our hike tomorrow.

Day #28
Day #2 Kerry Way
Hillcrest Farmhouse (Black Valley) to Glencar (Climber's Inn) –
13½ Miles
Total – 320 Miles

This morning, Day #2 on the Kerry Way, was the most beautiful day of this entire 28-day hike—at least the first half through the Black Valley. It was a long seven-plus-hour day of hiking, and our legs are beat. But the scenery was simply stunning.

I was up at 6am, and Leslie around 6:30am. It's the routine we've fallen into. I read the news, check emails, and, if there is still time, get some office work done. Leslie does news, emails, checks Facebook, and plays Wordle and Words with Friends on her iPad.

We were walking out of the Hillcrest Farmhouse a little after 9am, and within a few minutes, walked past the hostel in Black Valley. I assumed that we'd see other hikers today coming from the hostel, but we never met anyone on the trail going either direction until we were having a beer outside the Climber's Inn at the end of the day.

The Black Valley has high mountains rising up on both sides. There are a handful of sheep farms, but that is it. Quite remote. Spectacular scenery. Rocky mountains. The Gearhameen River. Cummeenduf Lough. The sun and clouds brought out a hundred shades of green in this incredible glacier-carved valley. If there was one day of hiking I would repeat some day in the future, it would be this second day on the Kerry Way.

There are apparently some rock-carved petroglyphs a few miles off-trail. There are also some standing stones and row stones that our guidebook says were put in place thousands of years ago when this area was the "center of life" in the region. Hard to imagine now with only the few scattered houses and stone walls for sheep.

We walked to the end of the valley along a narrow paved road, around a large sheep farm, and then straight up a rocky slope to a saddle that connects the Black Valley and the Bridia Valley. An ancient row of three large stones sits up on the saddle overlooking the valleys. The largest is about six feet tall.

It's so crazy to think that these massive stones were erected here, somehow, maybe 4,000 to 5,000 years ago! The view from the saddle into Bridia Valley was equal to the Black Valley view looking back the way we'd just hiked.

We took a lunch break around 12:30pm after taking a full three hours to hike only six miles. We could see hundreds of sheep scattered high up on the mountainsides, and ancient stone walls for livestock fences down below.

When the sun poked through the clouds, it was intense. The temperature was around 70 degrees with a breeze.

The downhill off the saddle was steep and rocky. I gave Leslie a good head start since rocky downhill hiking is not her forte. The remaining seven or so miles to Glencar seemed to take forever. The combination of heat, rocky ground, and the ups and downs of the trail took it out of us today. We were both downing Advil and dragging our tails the last few miles.

We met a farmer along the way moving a few dozen sheep by truck to a new area to graze. He said that the winters in Bridia are long, dark, and cold, so these rare warm summer days are really appreciated.

I filled our water bottles twice from little mountain streams, at spots where the water was moving fast over stones. I was hoping that there weren't enough sheep uphill to pollute the little streams with Giardia. I guess we'll find out. I remember hearing years ago that the best place to gather water for drinking is in a spot where the water has been moving quickly over rocks, rather than in places where the water is more stagnant.

Glencar consists of just the Climber's Inn. Nothing else there. But the inn has rooms, a small six-bed hostel, a pub that serves food, and a very small grocery store—everything a hiker on the Kerry Way needs to rest and restock.

Before even dropping our bags in our room, we had a beer outside at a picnic table. We'd both been dreaming about this beer for the last few hours. Leslie got a Harp Ale for the first time this trip, and I got my pint of Guinness.

As we drank our beer, two different cars pulled up and dropped off a total of three bedraggled hikers with big backpacks. Not sure where they came from. Another guy with a big backpack walked up to the inn, and then two bikers pedaled up about 30 minutes apart.

I've never seen bikers more loaded down with bags and gear. They seemed totally overloaded. The lady was covered in tatoos from head to toe and spent the hour that we stared at them spreading out her clothes, tent, sleeping bag, etc., to dry. (I'm not sure why, because it hasn't rained for days?) Meanwhile, the guy on the other bike talked non-stop, very loudly, and in French. We couldn't help staring at them the whole time, and thinking up scenarios of who they were, how well they did or did not know each other, and what was going on.

We only have three more hiking days!

Hard to believe.

I just moved our return flight up two days to July 20.

Day #29
Day #3 Kerry Way
Glencar (Climber's Inn) to Emirview B&B in Mountain Stage
near Glenbeigh – 11½ Miles
Total – 331½ Miles

Our Day in Four Parts:

<u>Part One:</u> Up and walking from the Climber's Inn by 9am. We walked back along the same kilometer we finished on yesterday to get back to the trail. It was really pleasant walking through shady forest. A few steep ups and downs, but almost all in the shade.

<u>Part Two:</u> Miles four through nine were hiked in the blazing sun. The entire U.K. and much of Europe are setting all-time high temperature records. On Monday, meteorologists are predicting the hottest day on record for this area. We literally watched a TV news reporter last night telling people to stay indoors.

We hiked up a long, fairly steep and exposed path to Windy Gap. We ate our lunch while appreciating the cooling breeze, then down, down, down to Glenbeigh while being passed by three speedy day hikers, all in their mid to late 70s.

<u>Part Three:</u> We were checked into our Emirview B&B by 2:15pm. I grabbed a quick shower just to cool off while Leslie popped a massive blister double the size of her little toe and taped it up. We left our packs at the B&B and hiked another two and a half miles just so tomorrow won't be as hard in the heat that is predicted to be worse than today.

This last part was a mostly shaded trail that wrapped around Drung Hill. The first part passed through a fairy forest filled with dozens of elaborate wooden fairy houses nailed to trees. We then caught a taxi ride from Mountain Stage back to our B&B.

<u>Part Four:</u> A great Killarney IPA at the Towers Restaurant on the main street of Glenbeigh. It's a cute little tourist town, and very busy on a sunny Friday afternoon in July. We had a nice, proper dinner. Leslie had pork, vegetables, and mash, and I had a grilled chicken breast with vegetables and mash.

Highlights of Our 11-and-a-Half-Mile Day:

- The fairy forest was cute, and it was fun to look at all of the brightly painted tiny houses. There were lots of tiny signs noting "fairy crossings" and asking for quiet during the day when the fairies are sleeping.

- As we came up over Windy Pass, after a grunt of an up-hill climb, we got our first views of the ocean that we've been heading towards for the past 29 days. Dingle Bay. We could also see most of the Dingle Peninsula from our high vantage point.

- After dinner at the Towers, we stopped at a SPAR store to buy snacks for tomorrow and I got a Snickers milkshake that I'd been dreaming about for quite a while. Leslie got a kiddie cone.

Low Points of Our 11-and-a-Half-Mile Day:

- Biting flies pestered us for most of the day, brought out by the heat.

- Leslie's feet have taken a turn for the worse.

Day #30
Day #4 Kerry Way
Mountain Stage near Glenbeigh to Cahersiveen's (Quinlan & Cooke Hotel) – 13½ Miles
Total – 345 Miles

Somehow, a planned 10- to 11-mile day turned into a 13-and-a-half-mile day. And my feet are not happy about it.

We asked our hostess at the Emirview if she could drive us back to where we left off yesterday afternoon, about two and a half miles past Glenbeigh at a spot referred to as Mountain Stage. After we finished an amazing breakfast of pancakes (crêpes) and bacon (ham), along with pure maple syrup from Canada (such a nice change from scrambled eggs), the owner's daughter had us to Mountain Stage by 9:15am.

The Kerry Way follows a rural road for one to two kilometers and then proceeds to climb up the side of Drung Hill, which is more of a mountain than a hill, for about a kilometer and a half. The trail was very rocky, and really challenged Leslie's aching feet and blister with every step she took. But as we climbed, the views of Dingle Bay were incredible. This part of the Kerry Way is another piece of an old "butter road," dating back to the late 1700s. The sun was as intense, or more so, than yesterday. It felt scorching hot by 9:30am.

In the 1700s, salted butter was an excellent way of capturing and preserving the natural nutrients that came through the cow's milk. However, much of this butter was produced far from the sea ports. The creation of these "butter roads" made it possible for a farmer to load up his horse with casks of butter for the market and make it there and back in two or three days, much quicker than following the old roads of the day. The butter casks where then shipped off to Holland, Spain, Portugal, and further afield.

We proceeded to roast in the sun all day long in temperatures that reached over 80 degrees. No clouds. No breeze.

After the Drung Saddle, the trailheads generally headed downhill and we had a little breeze to cool us off. But the heat made our feet swell and ache more than usual.

We each started the day with two liters of water and a liter of Gatorade. I ended up refilling our water bottles in little mountain streams, totaling two more liters each. We had finished them all off by the time we drug our exhausted asses into Cahersiveen. The sun really got to me today. We were both in a bit of a trance hauling our backpacks the last few miles on hot pavement with no shade.

The last seven to eight miles were, to be honest, miserable because of the heat.

Cahersiveen is a cute little town with lots of brightly painted old buildings, including several pubs along the main street. We are staying at the Quinlan & Cooke Hotel, and it's definitely the nicest (and most expensive) place we've stayed on this trip. Our room is large and has a bowl of fresh fruit and a small fridge with breakfast items.

We had dinner at Oratory Pizza and Wine Bar. Fantastic! A cool restaurant in a converted stone church.

Tomorrow is our last day!

We'll do it with only a daypack. It's supposed to be hot again tomorrow.

In some ways, the last 30 days have flown by. In other ways, it's hard to remember life before hiking.

Thirty straight days!!

Both of us feel like it was really no big deal.

But it is.

Getting up, putting on our packs, and going day after day after day isn't easy. And it's not always fun.

Our aging bodies have taken a bit of a beating on this long-distance hike.

Day #31
Day #5 Kerry Way
Cahersiveen to Bray Head on Valentia Island – 12½ Miles
Total – 357½ Miles

Day 31!

The final day of our cross-Ireland adventure.

The final day of a long-distance hike can be kind of anti-climactic. It's just another day of waking up, packing up, doing our morning stretches, putting on our packs, and walking out the door. (I was kidding about the stretching.)

Leslie's blister and feet still ache, and her limp was as pronounced as ever. I've been starting each day stiff and sore . . . right hip, knees, neck . . . until I get going.

I only carried a daypack today, which, as always, is way better than a full pack. But we still had 12 miles or so to get to the end of Valentia Island. Still a long way to walk.

The Kerry Way that we've been following for the past four days actually heads west a few miles before reaching Cahersiveen. We passed that turnoff yesterday. We continued on to Cahersiveen since the goal of this hike has been to walk across Ireland, leading to our ultimate destination on the western tip of Valentia Island. The full Kerry Way Loop is about 134 miles, and we just hiked the first almost half before turning off.

It was supposed to be hot again today. Predictions across Ireland and the U.K. were for all-time heat records. It turned out that it was 33 degrees Celsius in Dublin, and the all-time record was 33.3 degrees. That's a little over 91 degrees Fahrenheit. Plenty hot. In London, it was over 40 degrees Celsius, or 105 Fahrenheit! But there is no such thing as climate change or global warming, so that's a comfort.

For the first three miles walking out of Cahersiveen to the Valentia Island ferry, we walked through dense, cool fog. I knew it would burn off eventually, but I loved it while it lasted. As we got closer to the water and the ferry landing, I could smell the sea and started hearing seagulls squawking. We just couldn't see them. We could barely see any houses from the road because of the thick fog, and the few cars that passed seemed to sneak up on us.

We walked right on to the small, empty car ferry and then found out that the ferry had been waiting for over an hour for the fog to lift. We were the only passengers. It's only a 10-minute ride across to Valentia Island, but we couldn't see it through the fog until just before we docked on the other side.

Valentia Island is connected by a bridge to "mainland" Ireland on the other side of the island, but it still has the feeling of being an isolated island community. There is only one small village on the island, Knight's Town (where the ferry docks), with a single hotel—The Royal Hotel Valentia—a caravan park (campground), a couple of restaurants, and a few local businesses. The rest of the island is dotted with year-round and summer homes, a few B&Bs scattered about, and the only remaining active slate quarry in Ireland that produces "Valentia Slate."

All-in-all, Valentia Island is a sleepy, quiet place that in the fall and winter must be super sleepy, and super quiet.

We were able to get ahold of one of the two taxi drivers on the island. The other driver wasn't working today. The one lady that was driving said that she wouldn't be able to meet us at Bray Head (the most western tip of the island) until 3pm or 4pm. We got off the ferry around 9:15am, so we had six or seven hours to cover the remaining eight miles to the lookout tower at Bray Head, and then the one mile back to the car park.

We both did our best to enjoy and appreciate our final day. It was all road walking, except the final mile. There are basically two roads that lead from one end of the island to the other. We choose the road that follows the southern side of the island and hugs the coast, so we were near the water most of the way.

The sun eventually burned off the fog and the air heated up. Thankfully, we had an ocean breeze for most of the day.

We walked past several old stone houses whose slate roofs had caved in decades ago, and past several abandoned but not-for-sale houses that included one right on the water. It would make a perfect B&B location.

We started seeing the stone and concrete tower that sticks up at tip of Bray Head when we were still three or four miles away. That was the endpoint that I'd seen in lots of photos when I first started planning this hike. It was cool to be able to see the endpoint for the last hour or so.

Bray Head is a prominent rocky point that rises above the surrounding area and ends with dramatic cliffs that drop several hundred feet to the crashing ocean below.

Just before reaching the gravel car park and the start of the final mile of trail to the tower, we passed some remnants of old stone buildings that were the site of the first transatlantic telegraph station that sent the first electronic message by undersea cable from Europe to North America. According to the Internet, on August 16, 1858, Queen Victoria and U.S. President James Buchanan exchanged telegraphic pleasantries, inaugurating the first transatlantic cable connecting Ireland to North America. The Queen's 98-word greeting of goodwill took almost 16 hours to send through the 3,200-kilometer cable. Compared to 10 days by steamship, the cable was a tremendous improvement in speed for urgent communications.

We walked past a parking area that had a few dozen cars and started the final mile-long walk to the tippy end of Valentia Island, and the end of our 31-day hike. The last mile to the end was rocky and uphill the whole way, a final little test for our sore muscles and feet. There were dozens of tourists who were also making the one-mile hike from their car.

I remarked to Leslie that it's a weird feeling to know that no one knows that we just spent the last 31 days hiking across Ireland. We are walking this final mile up to the tower, just like they are, except for us this is the end of months of planning, anticipation, route finding, long and hard days of hiking, scores of helpful and friendly people we met along the way, our time hiking with "the kids" and Nora, Mary, Sean, John, Danny, and Olive, and on and on and on.

Everyone has their own route to travel, to get to where they are going.

Political discussions with taxi drivers.

Offers for rides that we turned down almost daily.

Pint after pint of perfectly poured Guinnesses.

Some rain.

Lots of sun and amazing weather.

Developing a routine of packing up every morning, where everything has its place and its purpose. Everything we carried, we either used or sent home weeks ago.

How many Advil and Tylenol?

How many rolls of medical tape and blister pads?

How many filled and consumed bottles of water?

How many maps and daily hiking notes and mileage markers to help us get where we are going?

How many earnestly sought and happily discovered trail signs to confirm that we were on the right route?

How many times we laced up our shoes in the morning and unlaced them to release our aching feet at night?

How many times did we rinse out our socks and shirts and underwear, and then drape them over light fixtures and window handles and door knobs to drip-dry?

How many pubs and restaurants and B&Bs and uncomfortable pillows?

How many audible sighs of relief as we eased into bed every night by 8pm to take the pressure off of our throbbing feet?

How many protein bars and handfulls of trail mix?

How many encouraging words of astonishment and disbelief when we told people that we started walking at the Temple Bar Pub in Dublin?

How many supportive emails and texts from our kids and our moms?

These are some of the reasons when people ask, "Why?"

Now, we're flying back across the ocean, two days after snapping photos on the cliffs at Bray Head with Leslie and Monkey Face, my adventure companions for the past 30 years. Thousands more memories, hundreds more stories, dozens more friends.

The world is mostly good.

Despite the raging war in Ukraine. Despite the Donald Trumps of the world. People are mostly good.

If life is truly "a daring adventure, or nothing," as Helen Keller once said, I'll choose the daring adventure every time.

- J.W.

EPILOGUE

9/05/15

(Years before we started our hike across Ireland, our hike around the coast of Wales, and my through-paddles of the Mississippi and Tennessee Rivers)

We all have stories to tell. And mine is much like everyone else's. But it is mine alone. I woke up this morning in a little bit of a panic, with my mind racing about things I still want to do before I die and about making a noticeable difference—leaving my mark on the world so that my time here wasn't a waste.

I'm feeling stagnant. Pretty bored. And it makes me want to act. Something big. Several somethings big. When all I can think of is moving to another country, and climbing a major mountain in South America, and building a log house from scratch in Colorado, and starting another long-distance adventure, I know it's time to do something.

It could be a little of my mild ADHD kicking in. I know it's not a mid-life crisis, though at 54 I'm at the perfect age for one. But I had a mid-life crisis when I was in my early 30s, and that felt way different. Then, I felt trapped and desperate and gasping for breath.

This isn't that.

Right now, what I'm feeling is more like super antsy with pent-up adventure energy, combined with bored. I'm ready to push myself into something unknown, into something that will really challenge me physically and mentally and emotionally. Into something that has the potential to change me.

APPENDIX ONE
Our Ireland Coast-to-Coast Itinerary

Wicklow Way

> Dublin to Clonegal
> 8 Days, 91.3 miles (11.4 mpd)

South Leinster Way

> Clonegal to Carrick-on-Suir
> 6 Days, 70.3 miles (13.5 mpd)

East Munster Way

> Carrick-on-Suir to Clogheen
> 4 Days, 40 miles (10 mpd)

Blackwater Way

> Clogheen to Clonkeen to Killarney
> 8 days, 93½ miles (11.7 mpd)

Kerry Way

> Killarney to Bray Head Loop on Valentia Island
> 5 days, 62½ miles (12.5 mpd)

Total Hiking: 31 days – 357½ miles (11.5 mpd)

June 15:   Depart Indiana 12:16pm

June 16:   Arrive Dublin 7:05am
                Lodging: Zanzibar Locke, Ha'Penny Bridge
                Check out Temple Bar Pub

Day 1:   Temple Bar to Morlay Park & Official Start -
                   5.5 miles
                Continue on trail to Pine Forest Art Center -
                   7 miles
                12.5 total miles for the day
                Lodging: Taxi to the "Firefly" in Bray -
                   9 miles

Day 2:   Taxi back to Pine Forest Art Center
                Pine Forest Art Center to Crone House Car Park -
                   8.4 miles
                Off-trail from Car Park to Coolakah House B&B -
                   1.8 miles
                10.2 total miles for the day
                Lodging: Coolakay House B&B

Day 3:   Got ride back to trailhead at Crone House Car Park
                Crone House Car Park to Wicklow Way Lodge
                   B&B - 11.5 miles
                Lodging: Wicklow Way Lodge B&B

Day 4:   Wicklow Way Lodge to Glendalough Lodge -
                   8 miles
                Lodging: Glendalough Lodge

Day 5:   Glendalough Lodge to Glenmalure Lodge in
                   Drumgoff - 10 miles
                Lodging: Glenmalure Lodge

Day 6:   Glenmalure Lodge to Kyle's Farmhouse B&B -
                    15 miles
                Lodging: Kyle's Farmhouse B&B

Day 7:   Kyle's Farmhouse B&B to Boley Bridge - 14 miles
                Got a ride B&B Owner to Shillelagh
                Lodging: Central House B&B in Shillelagh

Day 8:   Got ride back to Boley Bridge
                Boley Bridge to Clonegal - 10 miles
                End of Wicklow Way
                Taxi from Clonegal to Bunclody
                Lodging: Meadowside B&B in Bunclody

Day 9:   Taxi back to Clonegal
                Clonegal to Kildavin (Start of South Leinster Way)-
                    4.3 miles
                Kildavin to Cashell's Cross - 9.1 miles
                13.4 total miles for the day
                Got ride from B&B Owner to Boris
                Lodging: Brenda's B&B in Boris

Day 10:   Got ride back to Cashell's Cross
                Cashell's Cross to Graiguenamanagh - 11 miles
                Lodging: Waterside Guest House

Day 11:   Graiguenamanagh to Inistioge - 11.5 miles
                Lodging: Woodstock Inn

Day 12:   Inistioge to Mullinavat - 13.4 miles
                Lodging: Garrandarragh Inn in Rising Star

Day 13:   Mullinavat to Pilstown - 9 miles
                Taxi 5 miles to Carrick-on-Suir
                Lodging: Cariegh Hotel in Carrick-on-Suir

Day 14:   Taxi back to Pilstown
                Pilstown through Carrick-on-Suir to Kilsheelan -
                    12 miles
                End of South Leinster Way and Start of East
                    Munster Way
                Taxi to Clonmeal
                Lodging: Mulcahy's in Clonmel

Day 15:   Taxi to Kilsheelan
                Kilsheelan to Clonmel - 8 miles
                Lodging: Mulcahy's

Day 16:   Clonmel to Glasha Farmhouse (Four Mile Water) -
                    9½ miles
                Lodging: Glasha Farmhouse

Day 17:   Glasha Farmhouse to Clogheen - 12½ miles
                Lodging: Parson Green Caravan Park

Day 18:   Clogheen to Mountain Barracks - 10 miles
                Taxi to Mitchelstown
                End of East Muster Way
                Start of Blackwater Way
                Lodging: Clongibbon House in Mitchelstown

Day 19:   Taxi back to Mountain Barracks
                Mountain Barracks Fermoy - 10 miles
                Taxi back to Clongibbon House in Mitchelstown
                Lodging: Clongibbon House

Day 20:   Fermoy to Killavullen Loop Trailhead (Kilavulin) -
                    14½ miles
                Taxi to Mallow
                Lodging: Hibernian Hotel in Mallow

Day 21:   Taxi back to Killavulin

Killavullen Loop Trailhead to Ballynamona -
  10 miles
Taxi back to Mallow
Lodging: Hibernian Hotel

Day 22:   Ballynamona to Laharn Crossroads - 11½ miles
           Lodging: Donasheka House B&B

Day 23:   Laharn Crossroads to Mahon's Rock (Millstreet) -
             13 miles
           Taxi to Millstreet
           Lodging: Knockerish B&B in Millstreet

Day 24:   Taxi back to Mahon's Rock
           Mahon's Rock to Croohig's Cross - 11 miles
           Taxi back to Millstreet
           Lodging: Knockerish B&B in Millstreet

Day 25:   Taxi back to Croohig's Cross
           Croohig's Cross to Clonkeen - 12 miles
           End of Blackwater Way
           Taxi to Killarney
           Lodging: Failte Hotel

Day 26:   Taxi back to Clonkeen
           Clonkeen to Abbey Cross in Killarney - 11½ miles
           Taxi from Abbey Cross to Failte Hotel
           Lodging: Failte Hotel

Day 27:   Killarney (Abbey Cross) to Black Valley - 11½
             miles
           Start of Kerry Way
           Lodging: Hillcrest Farmhouse in Black Valley

Day 28:   Black Valley to Glencar - 13½ miles
           Lodging: Climber's Inn

Day 29:   Glencar to Mountain Stage (past Glenbeigh) - 11½
                  miles
               Taxi back to Glenbeigh
               Lodging: Emirview B&B in Glenbeigh

Day 30:   Taxi back to Mountain Stage
               Mountain Stage to Cahersiveen - 13½ Miles
               Lodging: Quinlan & Cooke Hotel

Day 31:   Cahersiveen to Valentia Island Ferry - 3 Miles
               Knight's Town to Bray Head - 9½ Miles
               Total for the day - 12½ Miles
               Ferry and taxi back to Cahersiveen
               Lodging: Quinlan & Cooke Hotel

APPENDIX TWO
List of What We Each Carried

- Backpack (Mountain Hardware Rocket)
- Lighter
- Sharp knife, spoon, and fork
- First Aid Kit: Advil, Band-Aids, blister pads, antibiotic ointment, Pepto bismol, anti-diarrhea pills, medical tape
- Hand soap
- Bandana
- Butt wipes
- Tooth brush, tooth paste, and floss
- Sunglasses and case
- Cellphone and charger
- Raincoat
- Rain pants
- Two extra undies
- Boxers for sleeping
- One extra pair hiking socks
- Two extra short-sleeve shirts (one for sleeping)
- Short-sleeve button shirt
- Long-sleeve button shirt
- Long-sleeve Lite PolyPro shirt
- One pair long pants
- One pair shorts
- Ear band and/or warm hat
- Two clothing stuff sacks
- Maps and guidebook
- Journal and two pens
- Small notepad
- Small drybag for map/computer case

- Headlamp and three extra batteries (AAA)
- Two one-liter water bottles
- Monkey Face
- Macbook Air and charger
- Waterproof pack cover
- Light down jacket
- Book
- Reading glasses
- Sanuks/Sandals
- Hiking Poles
- Hiking Shoes
- Packer hat

ABOUT THE AUTHOR

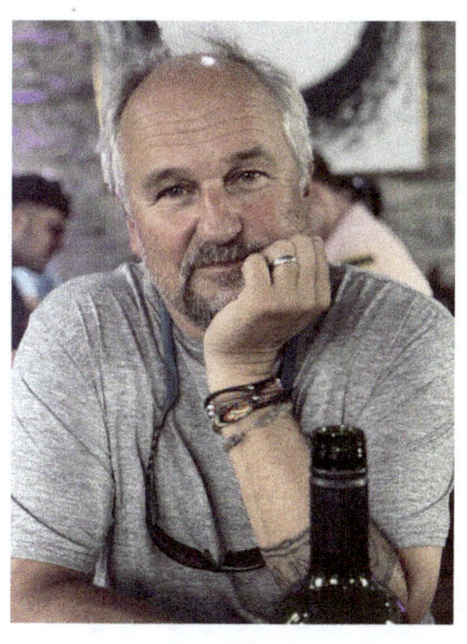

Author Jon Wunrow is the grateful grandparents of his grandchildren and future adventurers Arlo, Rio and Coletta; parent of amazing sons Seth and Tyler; and husband of his *anam cara* Leslie. Of much less importance, he is also a supporter of Ukraine, cabin builder, beer brewer, coffee roaster, grant writer, Tribal advocate, Green Bay Packer fanatic, and a dreamer, who occasionally finds time to plan and enjoy long-distance adventures around the world.

In addition to pursuing his passion for climbing most of the highest peaks in the Western Hemisphere, he has hiked the 2,650-mile Pacific Crest Trail, through-paddled the Mississippi and Tennessee Rivers as well as paddling seven weeks across Manitoba, and climbed Kilimanjaro with his son Seth. He and Leslie have also hiked the 870-mile Wales Coast Path, England's 630-mile Southwest Coast Path, and most recently hiked 357 miles across Ireland. In 2023, he and a friend bicycled across Mongolia.

Wunrow has also authored *Me and Sadie: We Got Everything We Need: Stories from Paddling the Tennessee River* (2022), *Paddling the Mississippi: One Story at a Time* (2022), *Never Stop Walking: A Wale's Coast Path Adventure* (2021), *High Points: A Climber's Guide to South America* (2018), *Adventure Inward: A Risk Taker's Book of Quotes* (2013), and *High Points: A Climber's Guide to Central America* (2012).